Occupational
Social Work Today

Occupational Social Work Today

Shulamith Lala Ashenberg Straussner
Editor

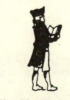

The Haworth Press
New York • London

Occupational Social Work Today has also been published as *Employee Assistance Quarterly*, Volume 5, Number 1 1989.

The Haworth Press, Inc. 10 Alice Street, Binghamton, NY 13904-1580
EUROSPAN/Haworth, 3 Henrietta Street, London WC2E 8LU England

Library of Congress Cataloging-in-Publication Data

Occupational social work today / Shulamith Lala Ashenberg Straussner, editor.
    p. cm.
    "Has also been published as Employee assistance quarterly, volume 5, number 1, 1989" —
T.p. verso.
    Includes bibliographical references.
    ISBN 0 – 86656 – 995 – 2. – ISBN 0 – 86656 – 998 – 7(pbk.)
    1. Welfare work in industry – United States. 2. Welfare work in industry. I. Straussner, Shulamith Lala Ashenberg.
HD7654.028   1990
361.7′65′0973 – dc20   89-27967
                                                        CIP

Occupational Social Work Today

CONTENTS

Social Workers' Role in Promoting Occupational Health and Safety

Beth M. Lewis

ABOUT THE EDITOR

Shulamith Lala Ashenberg Straussner, DSW, CEAP, is Assistant Professor at New York University School of Social Work. In addition to teaching, conducting research, and consulting to private industry and hospitals in the areas of employee assistance programs and alcoholism and drug addiction, Dr. Straussner is a certified psychoanalytic psychotherapist and has a private clinical practice in New York City.

Dr. Straussner is an active member of the Association of Labor-Management Administrators and Consultants on Alcoholism and the New York City Chapter of the National Association of Social Workers. She is on the Advisory Board of the chapter's Industrial Social Work Committee and a past president of the chapter's Committee on Alcoholism and Other Drug Dependencies. She has presented papers and conducted numerous workshops at various local and national conferences.

Dr. Straussner is the author of numerous publications and has edited several issues of the journal *Alcoholism Treatment Quarterly*. She is a co-editor of the book *Psychosocial Issues in the Treatment of Alcoholism* (The Haworth Press, 1985).

Preface

The field of Occupational Social Work is still in the process of defining itself. While the seven articles in this publication do not represent a comprehensive picture of occupational social work today, they do attempt to provide an in-depth discussion of some of the areas in which social workers find themselves, and to address some of the current issues which they encounter.

The first article by Straussner attempts to provide a historical context and a conceptualization of this still evolving field. The article by McCarthy and Steck aims to help social workers enhance their skill in assessing the corporate culture in which they may find themselves, while the article by Molloy and Burmeister attempts to sensitize workers to the unique nature of union-based social services.

One of the fastest growing areas in the field of occupational social work is managed mental health. Wagman and Schiff describe the evolution of managed health care and the roles and skills which are utilized by social workers working in this area.

One of the newest arenas in which social workers find themselves is human resource management. In his article entitled "Application of Social Work Skills to Human Resource Management," Philip Berry discusses the impact of the changing workforce on human resource and the value of applying social work skills in this area. Job loss is an issue which affects all level of employees from top management to factory workers. Foster and Schore describe the variety of ways in which social workers can help workers deal with the trauma that job loss evokes.

In the final article in this publication, Lewis discusses the importance of social work skills in the area of occupational health and disability. Although in comparison to other areas within the field of occupational social work there are few social workers who are dealing with occupational health and safety, this is certainly an area in which social work skills are highly applicable.

This publication attempts to present the state of the art of some aspects of the field of occupational social work. While social workers have moved rapidly into this new field, there is a need for many more social workers who are capable of combining good social work skills with the specialized knowledge needed in order to effectively function in the world of work and of workers.

Shulamith Lala Ashenberg Straussner

Occupational Social Work Today: An Overview

Shulamith Lala Ashenberg Straussner

SUMMARY. Over the last two decades we have seen a significant increase in social work interest and presence in the world of work. This article provides an overview of the growing field of occupational social work, discusses its historical roots, and presents a typology of five different service models which are currently provided by occupational social workers.

No other technique for the conduct of life attaches the individual so firmly to reality as laying emphasis on work: for his work at least gives him a secure place in a portion of reality, in the human community. (Freud, 1930: 27)

The focus of the social work profession has always been on the "human community." However, the workplace—the "crossroads of life" according to one of the pioneers of the profession, Bertha Reynolds (1975)—has frequently been an ignored component of this community. This is no longer true. Since the 1970s social workers, as well as other professionals, have rediscovered that the workplace is "not for work alone (but) . . . a unique and important site where employees can and should be informed about non-work related services and where actual diagnosis of selected needs and delivery of selected services can take place" (Spiegel, 1974: 31).

The current interest of social workers in the world of work and the increasing employment opportunities in this field are the conse-

Shulamith Lala Ashenberg Straussner, DSW, CEAP, is Assistant Professor, New York University School of Social Work, and is also an EAP and Substance Abuse Consultant. Mailing address: New York University School of Social Work, 2 Washington Square North, New York, NY 10003.

1

quences of the changing interplay of economic, political, social, demographic and legal forces over the last two decades. This combination of forces has pushed employers to provide a growing number of programs and services not only for those who are or have been employed, but also for their family members (Kamerman & Kingston, 1982; McGowan, 1984). Today's workers can receive employer- and union-sponsored assistance for a wide range of personal and social needs which benefit the young, the middle-aged and the old, and range from child care to pre- and postretirement counseling.

Many of the occupational services provided by social workers fall within the domain of traditional social work functions — such as direct counseling to employees. However, increasing sophistication of social work training in the emerging field of occupational social work, as well as in such areas as economics, policy analysis and planning, organizational assessment, research, and community development, combined with the contributions of a growing number of individuals with experience in the business world who chose social work as a "second career," make it a profession capable of functioning in such nontraditional social work areas as human resource and organizational development, corporate social responsibility and corporate philanthropy, and occupational social welfare benefit planning. Thus the relatively broad knowledge base of the professional social worker meshes with the complex needs of today's workplace.

This article provides an overview of the field of occupational social work, discusses its historical roots, and presents a typology of the current social work services and roles in this field.

DEFINITION AND ORIGINS OF OCCUPATIONAL SOCIAL WORK

Occupational social work can be broadly defined as a specialized field of social work practice which addresses the human and social needs of the work community through a variety of interventions which aim to foster optimal adaptation between individuals and their environments. In this context, the occupational social worker may address a wide range of individual and family needs, relationships within organizations, and the broader issues of the relationship of the world of work to the community at large (NASW, 1987). The occupational social worker utilizes social work knowledge, skills, and values to provide services, programs, and policy directions with and/or for workers and work organizations. As stated by Akabas (1983: 132): "the turf of occupational social work comprises those policy, planning and service delivery activities at the intersection of social work and the world of work." Among such activities are employee assistance programs, health promotion, managed health care, affirmative action, child and elder care, human resource development, organizational development, career development and training, work with the unemployed and those experiencing job retrenchment, corporate social responsibility, employee benefits, occupational health and safety, job development, pre- and postretirement planning, and relocation assistance (NASW, 1987).

While occupational social work is one of the newest fields within the social work profession, the historical roots of occupational or industrial social work in the United States date to the late 19th century "welfare capitalism" and the employment of "social secretaries" by private industry.

Welfare capitalism refers to those benefits and services provided voluntarily by employers in an effort to socialize, retain and control a raw unskilled and badly needed labor force at a time of rapid industrialization (Brandes, 1976). The antecedent of the employment of industrial social workers can be traced to the employers' attempt to deal with the problems resulting from the rapid increase of women in the labor force following the Civil War. According to Brandes (1976):

> The beginnings of industrial social work are rooted in what might well be considered a form of sexism . . . as businesses grew and employers faced growing numbers of female employees, they found themselves at a loss about treating their workers' peculiar "female" problems; one answer was the hiring of "specialists." Probably the first was Mrs. Aggie Dunn who was hired in 1875 as "social secretary" for the H.J. Heinz Company of Pittsburgh. (Brandes, 1976: 111)

Dunn was probably the only welfare secretary until 1900 when many other companies began hiring such specialists. A 1919 Bureau of Labor Statistics survey of 431 of the largest companies in the United States found that 141 companies employed a full-time welfare secretary, while—an interesting precursor of today's contractual or external programs—154 companies contracted with outside agencies for social work services. By 1926, 80 percent of the 1,500 largest companies in the United States had some type of welfare program (Popple, 1981).

Although by 1920 more graduates of the New York School of Social Work were employed in industrial settings than in any other area (Popple, 1981), professionally trained social workers were still few in number and most of the welfare secretaries were women educated as teachers or nurses. One such nurse, a Mrs. Marion T. Brockway, was hired as the "house-mother" at the Metropolitan Life Insurance Company. In announcing her appointment in the September 3, 1919 issue of the official publication of the company, Metropolitan Life's President Fiske described her duties as follows:

The House Mother's duties will be such as are involved in the title. Any female employee will be welcome to consultation as to her health, her work, her relations to her associates and superiors and her domestic relations, her personal affairs and worries, if any. Mrs. Brockway will look into the conditions of service in the office and will be glad to advise in case of difficulties inside or outside of the office, and as to residence and its surroundings and board of those who do not live with near relatives.

While primarily our idea of the appointment of a House Mother was our feeling that our female Clerks would appreciate her service, yet Mrs. Brockway will be only too glad to advise with any male Clerks to whom she can be of help. Her mature years, her wide experience, her gift of common sense, her capacity for sympathy, fit her to advise with men as well as women. And all our Clerks will be welcome to consult with her . . .

In general, the roles of welfare secretaries fell into four categories (Carter, 1977):

- Physical Welfare—which included responsiblities for the health, safety, sanitation and housing of workers;
- Cultural Welfare—which covered areas such as recreation, libraries, education and basic acculturation to the workplace and American values;
- Personal Welfare—which covered casework services for workers and their families; and
- Economic Welfare—which included administration of loans and pensions and even the hiring, firing and wage setting of employees. (Brandes, 1976)

Due to a combination of forces, including worker dissatisfaction, the changing economy, the increasing availability of services provided by the social work community, and shifting social ideology (see Straussner & Phillips, 1988), these early industrial social workers disappeared from industrial settings almost completely during the 1920s only to reappear during World War II as "social work services not only helped people adjust personally to the effects of the war but also enabled them to be more productive during a time when production was a critical common goal" (Masi, 1982: 6). At this time, social workers functioned as direct service providers in union settings (see Kyle, 1944; Reynolds, 1963), in the federal government and armed services (Stalley, 1944), and in a number of private firms such as Macy's in New York (Evans, 1944), RCA Victor in Indianapolis (Coyle, 1944), J. L. Hudson department store in Detroit, and Metropolitan Life Insurance Company (Palevsky, 1945).

The development of modern occupational social work is generally traced to the 1960s with the establishment of two separate programs aimed at addressing the mental health needs of workers. Both of these highly successful programs, one established by the management of the Polaroid corporation in Boston, and the other by the Amalgamated Clothing Workers of America in New York City, were directed by professional social workers (Kurzman, 1987). The subsequent spread and visibility of this newly emerging field can be credited to a large degree to the Industrial Social Welfare Center which was established in 1969 at Columbia University School of Social Work under the direction of Hyman J. Weiner and funded by the Social and Rehabilitation Service of the U.S. Department of Health, Education and Welfare. The aim of the Center was three-fold: To build a knowledge bank and to serve as a clearinghouse for information related to provisions of various social services to the working population; to provide technical assistance and consultation services to organized labor, business firms and community agencies; and to "influence" the education of social workers and other helping personnel (CUSSW, 1974). The Center has been largely successful in achieving its aim.

By the mid-1970s, "(t)he scatter-gun beginnings of industrial social work at the start of this century [had] developed into an organized movement" (Masi, 1982: 14). This development was the consequence of multiple forces including: the decrease of professional social workers' affiliations with the public sector; the increasing growth of private practice among social workers; the changing workforce due to the entry into the workplace of large numbers of women, minorities, and the disabled; the various work related legislations such as the Hughes Act, the Vocational Rehabilitation Act, the Occupational Safety and Health Act, the Employee Retirement Income Security Act, the Age Discrimination in Employment Act, and Title VII of the Civil Rights Act; and the increasing social awareness of the impact on the workplace of workers' mental health in general, and alcoholism in specific. Furthermore, the professionalization of the Occupational Alcoholism Programs and their evolution into Employee Assistance Programs combined with the establishment of occupational social work training programs in a number of schools of social work throughout the United States and Canada increased both the employment opportunities and the availability of trained social workers for these new positions.

While the exact number of occupational social workers today is unknown, the National Association of Social Worker compiled a mailing list of 2,200 individuals as part of their 1985 national survey of occupational social workers. As of 1987, 614 licensed social workers were members of the Association of Labor-Management

Administrators and Consultants on Alcoholism (ALMACA), the main professional organization representing those working in employee assistance programs (EAPs), and as pointed out by Googins (1987: 37): "social workers hold leadership positions and constitute far and away, the primary professional group" in occupational associations such as ALMACA, EASNA (Employee Assistance Society of North America), and the IASISW (International Association of Industrial Social Workers).

Occupational social workers today are employed in the private sector (both for-profit and voluntary), in the federal, state, and local levels of government, in the military, and in labor unions. A national survey of 39 schools of social work which offered occupation social work training indicated that 30% of their field placements were in private sector organizations, 23% with contractors providing services to companies, 17% in state, county or local government agencies, 15% in union and 15% in federal government agencies (Maiden & Hardcastle, 1985). While occupational social workers provide a wide variety of services in a wide variety of settings, the most common setting of occupational social service delivery today is through employee assistance programs (EAPs).

OCCUPATIONAL AUSPICES AND PROGRAM MODELS

In fulfilling the various occupational social work functions, the social worker may be employed under the auspices of a trade union, a peer group (an association of individuals in the same trade who are not necessarily members of an organized labor union), or the management of either a private or a public organization. In some, relatively few, instances, the auspice may be provided jointly by labor and management (see Straussner, 1986).

Occupational programs and services can also be sponsored through a single organization or firm, or through consortia in which several organizations pool their resources and jointly develop or sponsor a program. Another variable is the program model: In the in-house or internal model, the occupational social worker is directly employed by the organization (company or union) sponsoring this function, while in the contractual, also referred to as external or vendor model, the work organization or union makes a contractual arrangement with a self-employed social worker, a group practice, a private proprietary firm, or a voluntary agency to provide the needed services to the workers. For example, a self-employed occupational social worker can have a contractual arrangement to provide consultation services focusing on establishing a child care program which will be sponsored by a consortium of several organizations, while another social worker may be employed directly by a union to develop an in-house preretirement program for union members, and still another occupational social worker may be employed by a voluntary hospital that contracts with the management of several local businesses to provide external employee assistance programs to their employees, and a group of social workers may form their own entrepreneurial firm which provides outplacement services.

A TYPOLOGY OF OCCUPATIONAL SOCIAL WORKERS' SERVICES, ROLES, AND SKILLS

One way of conceptualizing the various services provided by occupational social workers and the roles and skills utilized by them is through a typology comprised of five models: the employee service model, the employer or work organization service model, the consumer service model, the corporate social responsibility model, and work related public policy model. This typology is an extension of the three-dimensional service approach—the employee service, the consumer and the corporate social responsibility models—developed at the University of Pittsburgh and elaborated by others (Johnston, 1983; Shank, 1985). While the typology is presented as consisting of five discrete components, in reality an occupational social worker may function in more than one model and assume a combination of roles at any one time. A detailed discussion of these models is presented below.

1. The Employee Service Model

This model focuses on implementing programs and providing services that, while benefiting either management by increasing worker productivity and commitment to the organization or unions by increasing or maintaining the workers' allegiance to the union, are primarily aimed at the needs of individual employees.

Within this model fall the variety of programs and direct services aimed at helping workers cope with the various physical, mental, familial and social problems which either directly or indirectly relate to their roles as workers. Included in this category are the variety of activities and services which fit into the domain of employee assistance programs (EAPs) and member assistance program (MAPs), as well as a wide range of occupational health prevention and wellness models such as stress management, smoking cessation, preretirement planning, and so on. While such services may be provided within a group setting, their aim is the well-being of individual employees.

The employee service model is the most common model utilized by occupational social workers and the one most likely to utilize traditional social work roles such as counselor, mediator, advocate and broker. A description of these roles and skills is provided below.

Counselor — in this role the occupational social worker provides assessment and short- and/or long-term counseling with individuals, families and groups. The social worker helps people to articulate their needs, to identify and to clarify their problems, to understand the possible dynamics or causes of their problems, to explore various alternatives and solutions, and to develop their capacities to deal with their own problems more effectively. The skills and knowledge base essential to this role are similar to that employed by social workers in other settings and include biopsychosocial assessment or diagnostic skills, interviewing skills, skills in assessment and intervention with individuals with a wide variety of psychopathology and stress reactions including drug- and alcohol-abusing individuals and/or their family members, crisis intervention skills, knowledge of counseling and communication skills, knowledge of group and familial dynamics, as well as understanding of economic realities. What makes occupational social work counseling different from social work counseling in other settings is the occupational social worker's need for systemic understanding of the world of work, their knowledge of the differential roles of management and labor, and the impact of the workplace on the functioning of the individual worker. For example, in seeing a female employee who was in job jeopardy due to excessive lateness and absenteeism, the union-based occupational social worker assessed that the reason for the worker's problem was not only her low level of self-esteem related to her traumatic childhood and her current feelings of depression and helplessness, but also her inability to deal effectively with the advances of a male co-worker. After further exploration of various options and with the support of the worker's supervisor and her shop steward, the social worker enabled the employee to ask for and obtain a transfer to a different department in the organization.

Constructive Confrontator — this is a unique role assumed by those trying to help individuals experiencing drug and alcohol problems. Due to the denial inherent in substance abuse, the traditional counseling roles assumed by social workers are usually ineffective in getting substance abusers into appropriate treatment (Levinson and Straussner, 1978), thus specialized confrontative or "interventve" approaches need to be utilized (Johnson, 1986). In this role, the occupational social worker may call upon the supervisor, union representatives, and family members to confront the substance abuser with the problems resulting from the abuse of alcohol or other chemicals and provide the employee with a prearranged treatment plan. A thorough understanding of the dynamics of substance abuse, family systems, authority issues and peer pressure are essential in fulfilling this role.

Broker — in this role the occupational social worker links individuals who need help with existing resources — both in and out of the company — that may be of service to them. For example, in helping substance abusing employees, the worker may refer an employee to an in-patient alcoholism rehabilitation facility, to the company medical department, or to a work- or community-based self-help group meeting. Included in the broker role is some form of systematic follow-up on such referrals. The skills and knowledge base inherent in this role includes knowledge of referral skills, understanding of individual and organizational resistance, knowledge of organizational and community resources, skills in advocacy of resource development, and networking skills.

Advocate — in this role the occupational social worker helps workers obtain services and resources which, due to a variety of causes, they have been unable to obtain on their own. This role, borrowed from the legal profession, is a highly active one in which the worker advocates on behalf of employees' needs and requests, provides leadership in collecting relevant data and in challenging institutions' decisions in order to modify or change current positions or policies. Although this role is less likely to be used in settings in which the occupational social worker is employed directly by private industry (Straussner, 1986), it is an important role undertaken by union-based social workers as well as by other occupational social workers.

Mediator—in this role the occupational social worker manages conflicts between two or more individuals or systems and interprets the needs of each to others. Skills include assessment of the nature and cause of conflict and creating a proper climate in which it is possible to effectively utilize such conflict resolution skills as identifying areas of commonality, separating problems from solutions, depersonalizing the situation, and examinating alternative solutions, (Johnston, 1983). It is a critical role in serving employees who may be referred involuntarily and helping to clarify the boundaries between disciplinary and treatment issues for such employees (Googins 1976).

Teacher/Trainer—in this role the occupational social worker provides information, explanations and expressions of opinions and attitudes, as well as models effective behavior and skills. Included in this role are the variety of wellness programs, such as smoking cessation and stress management.

2. The Employer/Work Organization Service Model

This model is aimed primarily at assisting the employer or work organization to identify and develop policies and services in relations to the workforce. In this model it is the organization which is the primary client and not any individual or group of employees. Examples of occupational social workers' roles encompassed in this model include consultation on such issues as the establishment of a work-based day care facility, provision of managed health care services, analysis of the impact of downsizing or reduction of the workforce on the organization, consultation on the establishment of appropriate affirmative action plan for women or minorities, or the development of a customer service training program for a bank.

As in the employee service model, the occupational social worker performing these tasks may be hired as an outside consultant or may be part of the in-house staff, perhaps in the human resource department. While less developed than the employee service model, the use of the employer service model, long established in western Europe (Googins, 1987), is increasing.

The roles and skills which are commonly used in the employer service model include:

Consultant — in this role the occupational social worker works with others to increase their abilities to understand various aspects of organizational and human dynamics and increase their skills in problem solving.

Evaluator/Analyst — in this role, the occupational social worker gathers information and assesses or evaluates organizational and environmental dynamics, policies or legislations and their impact on the organization. For example, the worker may assess organizational position in relation to legislation dealing with drug-free workplace and the implications for this organization of implementing random drug screening procedures.

Trainer — in this role, the occupational social worker functions as a teacher helping selected members of the organization become aware or sensitive to problematic aspects of the organization. Included in this role may be supervisory training aimed at helping supervisors recognize and respond to troubled employees, or become sensitive to behaviors indicative of sexual harassment on the job.

Program Developer — in this role, the social worker identifies and implements new programs which serve the needs of the workplace. For example, the worker may assess the need for and establish a program focusing on relocation assistance in a company which is anticipating a move to another community, or may establish a work-study program connecting a local community college with a company which has had problems attracting qualified employees.

3. The Consumer Service Model

This model focuses on the needs of the consumers of the workplace as oppose to employees or employers. For example, the occupational social worker may develop programs to identify and service the needs of elderly consumers of public utilities who may be in danger of having their utilities cut off for lack of payment resulting from their physical or mental deterioration.

Among the roles included in this model are counselor, program planner and developer, consultant, and advocate.

4. The Corporate Social Responsibility Model

This model focuses on identifying and assisting corporations to make a commitment to the social and economic well-being of the community in which they operate. Between 1979 and 1984 corporate contributions to local communities increased by $1.3 billion (Burke, 1987). This financial increase resulted in a corresponding increase in corporate staffs including the hiring of many social workers.

The titles and responsibilities of social workers in this model vary greatly. Among the titles held by workers in this model are: charitable allocations analyst, urban affairs advisor, corporate social responsibility director, community relations consultant, or community servicees coordinator. Responsibilities may include identifying and linking the organization with community leaders, evaluating requests for contributions of community groups and charitable organizations, conducting community needs assessments, and consulting and/or developing new services and programs. The roles and skills included in this model are: community analyst and planner, budget allocator, program developer, broker, advocate, and negotiator.

5. Work Related Public Policy Model

This model includes the formulation, identification, analysis and advocacy for those public or governmental policies, program and services which directly or indirectly affect the world of work.

An example may be an analysis of various occupational health benefits and services preferred within a given community, or an analysis of the implications of the aging of the national workforce and the various public policy options which may impact on both the needs of older employees and of the workplace, and/or advocacy of certain policies such as programs for the retraining of retirees to reenter the workforce (see Safford, 1988).

The skills essential for this model include policy planning and analysis, program development, advocacy, coalition building and networking.

THE FUTURE OF OCCUPATIONAL SOCIAL WORK

It is to be anticipated that the need for occupational social workers will continue and probably increase in the future. According to a recent article in the *New York Times*:

> Employers are starting to prepare for the work force of the 1990s with an array of family-oriented benefit programs that had long been resisted by corporate America. The decline in births in the 1970s is expected to produce intense competition for first time workers in the 1990s, and many will be women in their childbearing years. . . . Studies have shown that new workers of the 90s will have less emphasis on job security and more on personal values . . . they believe in the importance of balancing their work and family lives. (Collins, 1988: 1, 12)

Given their training, which emphasizes a generalist systemic perspective and a multi-dimensional appreciation of individual and larger systems, occupational social workers are capable of helping individuals balance the world of work and the world of the family. They can help workers deal with such issues as child care, parenting leaves, housing and relocations, substance abuse, elder care, preretirement planning, dealing with occupational hazard, job loss and the myriad of other problems experienced by the workers of today and tomorrow. Occupational social workers can also help employers examine various organizational and human dynamics and social policies impacting on the world of work.

Given the world in which we live, occupational social workers will need to continue their increasing sensitivity to various cost accounting and quality control measures such as managed care and utilization review. They will also need to continue to struggle with some of the dilemmas inherent in being in this profession, such as "how to balance clinical or individual needs with environmental and organizational factors which directly or indirectly contribute to individual problems" (Googins, 1987: 45), and how to protect client confidentiality and live up to the profession's code of ethics while functioning in a host environment which is not always supportive or understanding of such values.

Social workers will also continue to struggle with such issues as the need for specialized professional preparation and their connection with such developments as the newly instituted Certified Employee Assistance Professional certification. They will also need to continue to address the never-ending issues of professional boundaries, professional identity and interdisciplinary relationships.

Over the past two decades we have seen a convergence between employers' concern for the social and psychological aspects of employees and the social work profession's interest in and ability to meet those needs (NASW, 1987). The profession has discovered that it is capable of helping not only the individual worker, but also the employer and the work organization while keeping in mind the impact of social policy on those in the world of work.

As the world of work changes so will the knowledge and contribution of social workers as well as the issues, dilemmas, and the challenges that will arise.

REFERENCES

Akabas, S. H. (1983). "Industrial Social Work: Influencing the System at the Workplace" in Dinerman, M. (Ed.) *Social Work in a Turbulent World*, Silver Spring, MD: NASW.

Brandes, S. D. (1976). *American Welfare Capitalism*. Chicago: The University of Chicago Press.

Burke, E. (1987). "Corporate Social Responsibility" in *Encyclopedia of Social Work, 18th Edition*. Silver Spring, MD: NASW: 345-351.

Carter, I. (1977). "Social Work in Industry: A History and a Viewpoint." *Social Thought*, 3(1): 7-17.

Collins, G. (July 20, 1988). "Wooing Workers in the 90's: New Role for Family Benefits." New York Times: 1, 14.

Columbia University School of Social Work (May, 1974). "The Industrial Social Welfare Center: What We Are," *Industrial Social Welfare Center Newsletter.* 1(1): 1, 5.

Coyle, E. J. (January 1944). "A Description of Industrial Counseling." *The Compass*: 16-19.

Evans, E. (January, 1944). "A Business Enterprise and Social Work" *The Compass*: 11-14.

Freud, S. (1930). *Civilization and Its Discontents.* Strachey, Trans., London: Hogarth Press.

Googins, B. (1987). "Occupational Social Work: A Developmental Perspective." *Employee Assistance Quarterly*, 2(3): 37-54.

Googins, B. (1976) "Industrial Social Work" in Ross, B. and Khinduka, S. (Eds.) *Social Work Practice*, Silver Spring, MD: NASW.

Johnston, N. (1983) "Social Work in Industry: Education for Practice in the Work Place" paper presented at Council of Social Work Education APA Meeting, March 13-16.

Johnson, V. (1986). *Intervention.* Minneapolis, MN: Johnson Institute Books.

Kamerman S. B. & Kingston, P. W. (1982). "Employer Responses to the Family Responsibilities of Employees," in Kamerman, S. and Haynes, C. (Eds.) *Families that Work: Children in a Changing World.* Washington, DC: National Academy Press.

Kurzman, P. (1987) "Industrial Social Work (Occupational Social Work)" in *Encyclopedia of Social Work, 18th Edition.* Silver Spring, MD: NASW: 899-910.

Kyle, C. (1944). "Case Work in Unions." *Proceedings of the National Conference of Social Work. 71st Annual Meeting.* New York: Columbia University Press.

Levinson, V. & Straussner, S. L. A. (1978). "Social Workers As Enablers in the Treatment of Alcoholics." *Social Casework*, 59(1): 14-20.

Maiden, R. P. and Hardcastle, D. A. (Oct. 1985). "Occupational Curriculum Development in Graduate Schools of Social Work" unpublished paper.

Masi, D. A. (1982). *Human Services in Industry.* Lexington, MA: D.C. Heath and Co.

McGowan, B. G. (1984). *Trends in Employee Counseling Programs.* New York: Pergamon Press.

NASW (1987). *National Survey of Occupational Social Workers.* Silver Spring, MD: NASW.

Palevsky, M. (1945). *Counselling Services for Industrial Workers.* New York: Family Welfare Association of America.

Popple, P. R. (1981). "Social Work Practice in Business and Industry 1875-1930." *Social Service Review*, 55(2): 257-269.

Reynolds, B. C. (1975). *Social Work and Social Living.* Washington, DC: NASW.

Reynolds, B. C. (1963). *An Uncharted Journey*. New York: Citadel Press.

Spiegel, H. (1974). *Not for Work Alone: Services at the Workplace*. New York: Urban Research Center, Hunter College of City University of New York.

Shank, B. (1985) "Considering a Career in Occupational Social Work?" *EAP Digest*, July/Aug: 54-62.

Safford, F. (1988) "Value of Gerontology for Occupational Social Work." *Social Work*, 33(1): 42-45.

Stalley, M. (January, 1944), "Employee Counseling in the Federal Service." *The Compass*: 20-22.

Straussner, S. L. A. (1986) *Helping Troubled Employees: An Analysis of Selected Employee Assistance Programs Under Management Auspices*. Doctoral Dissertation, Columbia University. Ann Arbor, MI: University Microfilms International.

Straussner, S. L. A. & Phillips, N. K. (March, 1988). "The Relationship Between Social Work and Labor Unions: A History of Strife and Cooperation." *Journal of Sociology and Social Welfare*, X(1): 105-118.

Social Work in Private Industry: Assessing the Corporate Culture

Dolores E. McCarthy
Sarah B. Steck

SUMMARY. Assessment is a generic social work skill applicable in a range of practice settings. As social workers move into industry and, in particular, into the corporate world, these assessment skills must be adapted to fit the environment. Recognition of the uniqueness of the corporate environment is essential. This article presents the nature of assessment in the corporate setting, focusing on the Employee Assistance Program. It looks at corporate culture, develops a dynamic assessment model, and offers applications to both organizational and clinical areas. The highlight is on the interplay of the levels in systems involved.

You are a social worker, an MSW, with a range of clinical and administrative skills, and an interest in occupational social work. Imagine yourself being approached by the Vice President of Personnel of a large company, such as a bank, a consumer goods firm, a high-tech computer company, an advertising agency, a communications organization or a manufacturing concern. The company is interested in potentially starting an Employee Assistance Program. What factors would you consider? What would you assess?

Dolores E. McCarthy, MSW, MS, is an EAP Consultant. Mailing address: 56 Seventh Avenue, New York, NY 10011. Sarah B. Steck, MSW, ACSW, is President of Steck Associates. Mailing address: 6002 32 Street, NW, Washington, DC 20015.

Both authors were formerly Directors of the Employee Consultation Service at CBS, Inc.

In the world of business, social workers are now recognized as professionals with special skills. The burgeoning of Employee Assistance Programs (EAPs) has provided the forum in which social workers have joined and, in fact, become a part of an unfamiliar culture. The skills which we may take for granted are often highly valued in the business environment. Our work in EAPs provides a needed service to business, and we also become role models in all our interactions with employees and managers.

Employee Assistance Programs are but one form of social work practice within the corporate structure. However, they form the sphere of practice that many corporations are most ready to accept. As EAPs expand and develop, growing numbers of social workers are employed in in-house positions and external consulting firms. The social work and management literature and the literature of allied professions is rapidly compiling collections of articles on this topic (Klarreich, 1985; Straussner, 1988; etc.).

AN ASSESSMENT MODEL

The cornerstone of the social work profession is the ability to assess the "person-in-situation." A strength of the social work profession, with its broad interdisciplinary base, is its ability to handle large-scale, multi-system assessment. Social work is especially strong in its capacity to combine an understanding of individual and environmental issues.

As an EAP social worker, your client is an individual member of a larger organizational system. Your client is also the corporation, whether you are an in-house Employee Assistance Program professional or an outside consultant hired to run or work with the EAP. Assessment, therefore, will occur within the individual and the organizational system, and will include an awareness of the influences of one system upon the other. It is an interactive model.

One of the salient principles of social work assessment centers upon "staying where the client is," and responding to needs and concerns as perceived by the client. This focus involves many skills, among them listening, empathy, and continuous evaluation of the person and the situation. In traditional mental health settings, social workers use their finely honed listening and assessment skills routinely; many, in fact, incorporate these skills into their sense of themselves and their daily lives.

Organizational development and occupational mental health are growing subspecialties. Our organizational and clinical knowledge has been evolving in its applications to the workplace as a social system (see McCarthy, in press). Value issues underlie the development of this knowledge.

Of particular importance are: the effects of business and corporate values on assessment, the concept of consumerism, and the dual-client relationship of the social worker to both employer and employee.

Social workers must apply their skills in response to a specific practice environment, retaining the objectives of the profession while recognizing the needs of the organization. In a corporate environment, particular values form the fabric of the system. The social worker, using assessment skills, considers three levels: environmental variables, (physical situations, ambient stresses and values outside the organization); the corporate system (organizational issues); and issues specific to the individual client (clinical issues).

All elements in the assessment system, including the environment, are fluid and dynamic. Even global political/economic issues affect the operations of an organization. A multinational economy affects industry in areas such as profits and loss, planning and development, marketing, management, production and finance. These in turn affect human resource issues such as hires, fires, layoffs, transfers, work pressures and other factors that have some impact on the lives of individual workers.

Conversely, individual workers bring their personal characteristics to the work environment. A range of intrapsychic and interpersonal issues including personality factors or difficulties such as emotional problems, substance abuse, family issues and marital crises directly and indirectly affect the workplace.

Social workers are very familiar with the use of assessment skills at many levels. We know how to consider a range of factors and are flexible enough to include these factors when making a decision.

The purpose of this paper is to explore how social workers apply these already developed skills in the corporate world.

CORPORATE CULTURE

In order to effectively direct or work in an EAP, a social worker must understand the corporate culture. By corporate culture we mean to convey how it feels to work in that company: how people and profits are managed, the hidden agendas of the company, the unwritten rules, and the norms which employees have come to accept. Deal and Kennedy (1982), in their work *Corporate Cultures*, define four elements of corporate culture: the business environment; values; heroes and rites, and rituals. To these we add the nature of the industry, employee demographics, and the corporate perception of people and people problems. Employee perception of the culture may vary whether the individual works at headquarters or in a plant; whether the employee likes the work, and whether he/she is able to satisfactorily balance work and family pressures. Culture is what each employee experiences in being a part of that particular business environment. While culture is often intangible and subtle, it is a tremendously significant force in the organization.

We concur with Deal and Kennedy (1982), in their view that values are the "bedrock" of corporate culture. It is the values and beliefs, spoken and unspoken, to which social workers must be sensitive in running an EAP. We must be particularly attentive to the company's bottom-line values. Many companies truly believe in EAP tenets. Others, in the end, see the EAP as not important to corporate mission. Of all aspects of corporate culture, values may be the most difficult to fully evaluate. The values which the EAP social worker espouses must exist independently of corporate values, particularly in the area of confidentiality. However, the social worker is in a unique position to subtly influence organizational values through modeling behavior, training efforts and workplace interventions. It is realistic to expect that the EAP will be fully accepted in the workplace only after it is well established and conflicts have been faced and resolved.

The EAP social worker might well be part anthropologist. Using the techniques of "participant observation," the social worker assesses the values of the culture and the behavior of the individuals within the culture.

Assessment of corporate culture begins when the EAP social worker first interacts with the corporation. This assessment will include talking to line, staff, union and management; observing the work environment and employee-manager interactions, and becoming aware of communications and values within the organization. To run an effective EAP, the social worker must make the EAP compatible with the environment without sacrificing professional values, and while remaining aware of organizational politics. As Nahrwold points out:

> Every business culture has both healthy and pathological aspects, and counselors should have the wisdom and professional distance to know which is which. . . . Effective staff members are able to "blend in" with their organization's culture and dress, affirming the positive, remaining critical of the negative, and effecting change in a manner that is both charitable and discreet. (Nahrwold, 1983, pg. 111)

Listening well and being continuously aware of the environment will enable social workers to accomplish this.

Corporate Structure

Social workers must understand the corporate structure in order to create a "fit" between the EAP and the organization. The physical location of the EAP is critical. Understanding how medical, human resources, personnel or outside consultants are viewed by management and line workers alike will influence the location and administration of the program. The geographical arrangement of the company and whether it is centralized or decentralized must be noted and evaluated. For example, locating an EAP in a medical department is effective when the medical department is strong and well-respected. In a different organization and culture, a location in the human resources or employee benefits office may be more appropriate. At times, an outside EAP consultant/vendor best fits corporate style. Regardless of the location, the social worker must emphasize the confidential nature of the program.

The director must run the EAP in a manner that is compatible with the company's structure or which is congruent with the way the company operates to encourage employee utilization. One must be aware of, and at times make concessions to organizational roles already well-established within the structure. These might include using regional representatives and taking advantage of the highly significant role of labor unions. Getting a sense of the "informal" aspects of the structure is often difficult for any newcomer into a company. Talking with labor leaders, as well as management, will provide one perspective. Most successful EAPs include both labor and management employees, setting an example for a more effective relationship between labor and management.

Once familiar with the corporate culture and structure, the social worker is able to formulate policies and training tailored to that organization.

Organizational Change

In order to make a contribution to the health of the entire corporation, the EAP social worker must be able to understand both the systems and "bottom-line" issues for the corporation. The EAP social worker often has a unique picture of corporate issues. This picture emerges from employee interviews, training and educational seminars, consultation with managers, and interaction with other company professionals. The confidential nature of many of these interactions often enables the social worker to be aware of what occurs in the corporation from a number of perspectives.

The EAP social worker may then be able to devise strategies to address some problems, or engage other company professionals such as organizational development and management development specialists in doing so. In addition to addressing existing difficulties, the social worker can also do presentation activities, such as management consultation and small group training.

As Diana Chapman Walsh put it:

> For the future, while EAPs that are oriented principally toward organizational effectiveness or productivity continue to administer emotional first-aid to employees they scoop out of the rapids, they should also move upstream in search of explanations for why so many tumble in. . . . Where conditions of

work exacerbate or cause employee problems, even where social supports in the workplace might be bolstered to buffer the
stresses of everyday life, here lies the future terrain of prevention, health promotion and enhancement of the potential of
working men and women. (Walsh, 1982, pg. 514)

Some of these conditions of work might be inadequate or unreal-
istic policies related to work and family, areas of weakness in managerial leadership, or excessive stress in the workplace, to name
only a few. The results of work situations would include myriad
problems for employees, managers and organizations alike. These
include work and family conflicts, ineffective management, and un-
derproductive employees. There are a number of avenues in which
the social worker can intervene. Managing work-family problems
and contributing to a better work environment are two such avenues.

In a landmark study, Burden and Googins (1987) looked at balancing job and homelife in two major corporations. They examined
such issues as the impact on employees of balancing work and family, how employees handle work and family responsibilities, and
how family responsibilities overlap with the workplace. Burden and
Googins found that there was a striking difference in the studied
employees' perceptions about corporate sensitivity to their needs in
the work and family area, even though the two companies are similar in terms of benefits, programs and policies. As they report,

> What is different is a more intangible set of messages that are
> transmitted through corporate culture which in one company
> communicates a sensitivity and in the other more of an insensi-
> tivity. This finding suggests, in part, that overall management
> and corporate policy and style can go a long way in projecting
> concern and sensitivity to working parents. (pg. 51)

The EAP social worker is in a strong position to influence employee perception of corporate concern, as well as to provide concrete services which address work and family problems. Through
sensitive listening and interventions, openness, and a willingness to
tackle difficult work and family issues, the social worker will be
contributing to the well-being of employees and to fostering a caring corporate culture. In addition, the social worker can offer spe-

cific individual and managerial consultations, child and elder care referrals, educational seminars, and resources for coping with work and family problems.

A second avenue in which the EAP social worker can make a significant contribution to unhealthy conditions of work is through helping to build a better work environment. Robert H. Rosen remarks that,

> During the 1990s, we can expect to find social workers all over the corporation teaching their business colleagues the value of people and productivity in the new "healthy company." These companies will know well the full value of human capital. Their innovative policies and programs will help to create new kinds of jobs, and exciting work partnerships that will benefit employees, their companies and their families. (Rosen, 1988)

EAP social workers can teach about the value of people not only as a role model through their actions, but also through the kinds of policies and programs which they recommend to the corporation.

Manager Training

For some programs, just getting the employee to the EAP is a major hurdle. Careful training of managers and union supervisors is critical to overcoming that obstacle. In designing the training sessions, a thorough assessment of the managerial and union population is essential: management and union culture, skills level, receptivity and perceived place in the organization must be understood. Social workers may undervalue the importance of their effectiveness at listening and interviewing as assessment skills. But these skills are very important, and often unavailable, in the business organization. In training managers to utilize the EAP, social workers must overcome what Tuechter and Utne (1982) call the phenomenon of "manager reluctance": the unwillingness of managers seemingly fully committed to their jobs, to perform such essentials as salary reviews and correcting below-standard performance. EAP training and consultation often focuses on this managerial reluctance to conduct the work performance discussion or approach a troubled employee. This reluctance often leads to enabling and lack of effective managing by an otherwise caring and competent manager. The social worker quickly learns to assess this in the course of EAP consultations, so that "manager reluctance" remains a theme in many aspects of training and consultations. Our approach to supervisory training utilizes social work expertise in empathic listening. This task is to hear the concerns, doubts and strengths of managers as we assess how best to support them.

CLINICAL ISSUES

We have discussed why the range of social work skills, and in particular, the skill of assessment, are valuable in a corporate setting. The clinical assessment process is enhanced because the social worker has a unique understanding of organizational culture, and its impact on the individual assessment.

The clinical assessment of employees considers factors included in all psychosocial evaluations: identifying data, presenting problems, current situation, brief history, diagnosis and recommendations. However, because of the nature of the EAP service delivery system and the client's expectations of the social worker in this system, certain clinical issues may be prominent within the corporate setting. These include: career/work-related issues, job performance and managerial referrals, alcoholism/substance abuse, financial/legal problems, and special populations, such as minorities and women.

Generally, employees do not see themselves as "patients" or "mentally ill" when seeking services of EAPs. Rather they present themselves as healthy adults requesting consultation for personal problems. They are likely to regard the EAP social worker as a "problem-solver," and tend to present a specific problem. They may or may not be "psychologically minded." The social worker's task in the assessment is to facilitate the problem-solving process, a characteristic of business itself, and to introduce recommendations for treatment.

Career/Work-Related Issues

The corporate setting emphasizes a particular social role, that of employee as client. In traditional social work practice settings, the client is viewed primarily within an interpersonal context, most often as a parent, spouse, family member or in a role which involves relationship to another person. Certainly, many referrals to the EAP are generated by such interpersonal or family situations. In the EAP, however, we also consider the client's relationship to work itself, as well as his/her relationship to management, union, subordinates and peers. Recent literature has begun to address this role. For example, Cohen and McGowan (1982) outline areas such as work history, current position (occupation, hours, salary, fringe benefits), job responsibilities, performance, autonomy and control, relationship with colleagues, supervisors and subordinates, work strains and satisfaction, career goals and self-concepts as a worker which are important in assessing an employee. In the area of "work organization," factors such as size, location, ambiance, organizational structure, opportunities and constraints are considered. In the interface between work and family, authors address issues such as mesh between work time and family time (shifts, hours, overtime, etc.), income, intrusion of work roles and responsibilities in family life and vice versa, work role and the expectations of significant others (including family of origin) and leisure activities.

Knowledge of career development theory, vocational psychology, economics and political theory, and industrial/organizational theory can assist the occupational social worker in addressing these variables in the clinical assessment. This knowledge can aid in gathering data, interviewing, and forming a diagnosis.

Job Performance/Managerial Referrals

Referral of individuals specifically because of job performance problems is unique to EAPs. As we know, research has shown that poor job performance can be caused by numerous factors including substance abuse problems, family and marital issues, emotional difficulties, depression, psychosis or medical problems. Because of the dual-client relationship of the social worker to both employer and employee, the assessment is complex. A psychosocial assessment includes an understanding of the individual employee, the corporate structure and the interactions between the two.

The assessment will cover the nature of the performance problem, status of disciplinary action, additional organizational or departmental stresses, the employee's relationship with the manager, and confidentiality. If substance abuse and other clinical problems are ruled out, organizational assessment will explore the possibility that the manager or the department may be the source of the problem. This organizational dimension adds to the complexity of the typical clinical assessment and requires a systems orientation. A thorough clinical evaluation, therefore, involves examining sociological and organizational norms and behaviors as well as intrapsychic factors when job performance is an issue.

Alcohol/Substance Abuse

Since EAPs have evolved out of occupational alcoholism programs, knowledge of alcoholism and drug abuse holds a special importance for the occupational social worker. Because the consumption of alcohol and other drugs, including prescription drugs, remains a major workplace problem, a psychosocial assessment should give particular attention to substance use or abuse. Awareness of substance abuse and other addictive behavior, such as gambling and eating disorders, is a routine aspect of every EAP assessment.

Financial/Legal Concerns

Most multi-service social work settings help clients with financial and legal concerns. However, within the EAP, these same concerns have additional implications. Work itself is essentially an economic activity and personal work-related concerns may surface in the workplace. Employees often use the EAP for problems with budgeting, over-extension of credit, planning for retirement, relocation, and so on. In addition, serious financial problems related to compulsive gambling, substance abuse, or embezzlement of corporate funds, may be brought to the EAP. Many clients, particularly younger workers, may be in serious debt and ashamed to admit this. The EAP social worker assesses the issues "behind" the financial concerns. Specific legal issues also handled by the social worker may include possible discrimination, sexual harrassment, legalities of substance abuse problems, threats of homicide and suicide, medical compliance, and disability. These must be addressed in a clinical assessment.

Specific Populations

Within the EAP, as within the work site, particular groups of employees may deserve special note. Women and minorities for example, hold certain social roles within the organization. These individuals experience unique stresses that affect their job expectations and performances. Other groups, such as the handicapped, the recovering substance abuser, the single parent and the dual-career couple are all subject to additional stress. Moreover, the EAP social worker develops knowledge of stresses relative to job category: shift work, high-tech work, employee subject to frequent travel or relocation, the unsupervised sales force, the "creative" employee, the union employee, the senior-level executive, the new-hire, the "dead-end" employee, and the preretirement worker. Further, employees subject to layoffs are a growing group. Clinically as well as organizationally, these issues influence the assessment process.

CLINICAL INTERVENTION

One of the purposes of the social work assessment is to determine what intervention will best bring about change. As certain characteristics of the corporate culture influence assessment, they likewise are reflected in recommendations for intervention. Problem-solving is likely to be the orientation of choice in the EAP relationship. As the business culture emphasizes economic concerns, so the EAP social worker will choose interventions that are of high quality and cost effective. This bottom-line mandate is reflected in the orientation of the organization, which is likely to support treatment through insurance reimbursement, occasionally subsidizing brief therapy within the EAP. In addition, many clients have a "problem-solving" orientation and may feel more comfortable with brief, problem-focused treatment. When required, of course, long-term treatment is recommended.

And when organizational intervention such as management consultation, small group discussion, training seminars and similar programs are requested and appropriate, again a goal orientation is needed. Both the organization and the individual client are "consumers of EAP services." This consumer-oriented perspective, balanced by professional values and ethics, reinforces the need for expert assessment and intervention recommendation. Recent trends in health care cost containment and management health care support this view.

USE OF SELF

Within the corporate setting, the social worker also assesses how to make "use of self," to be as flexible and responsive as the organization demands. Adaptation to corporate culture, including dress, use of language, observance of social customs, and participation in corporate functions influences the social worker's integration into the company and perhaps even the effectiveness of the clinical interventions. However, maintaining a sense of professional integrity helps the social worker cope with the stresses created by the dual client relationship. Ideally, the practitioner, assessing the organization's culture, "joins with" the individual employee in assuming certain values, yet pays equal attention to the needs of the organization. For example, if a client is having difficulties with a job supervisor, the social worker will assess the role, personality and style of the supervisor, the social climate and daily operations of the client's department, as well as organizational goals. In addition, the social worker will evaluate the client's personal characteristics. Equipped with this information, the social worker will be better able to assess the client/supervisor relationship and struggle—including the contributions of the client, the corporate/political issues, and the perceptions and expectations of and by the client in the work setting.

As part of the assessment, the social worker will observe how the client perceives the EAP as well as his/her relationship to the social worker. In self-referrals a greater degree of trust may be expected than in managerial referrals. However, the client's positive or negative perception of the work environment, and of authority, will influence the degree to which the social worker's expertise is accepted. A client's expectations and fears, such as "saving my job"; "looking good to my boss"; or "being afraid other people might find out I consulted the EAP," will affect the ongoing clinical relationship, and must be addressed in the assessment. The social worker, then, portrays a "self" that is concerned with the needs of the individual client, yet within the context of the organization.

COST CONTAINMENT

The EAP social worker must be increasingly aware of corporate issues such as cost containment and benefits issues. In the past, EAPs have tried to provide the best referral for a problem, regardless of cost. For instance, a substance abuser is most often referred to a twenty-eight day inpatient treatment center. While this may be the appropriate treatment, the costs are staggering. The EAP social worker must be willing to explore treatment options which are both good for the client and acceptable to the organization, while never sacrificing quality. Similarly, the EAP social worker must work closely with the benefits department to ensure that the benefits provided are consistent with the health and mental health needs of the population.

In addition, an EAP program can ultimately influence some community treatment resources. The impact of the EAP social worker on community services is usually strong. The EAP referral process changes the nature of these services because the organization demands cost-effective treatment modalities. The assessment process expands to include the EAP's awareness of the values and culture of agencies and community services which accept referrals.

PROGRAM EVALUATION

The effectiveness of the EAP, both organizationally and clinically, must also be assessed. Although practical constraints often impede formal research-oriented evaluation, certain principles can be applied to monitor the program and services delivered.

Evaluation of the EAP and its impact on the corporation is essential. Formal evaluation methods include daily statistics, assessment instruments, and personnel supervision. Follow-up questionnaires with employee and manager usually reveal how the EAP's intervention helped the employee, as well as the satisfaction of the family, the co-worker and/or manager/union representatives. A computer can be a great help in the analyzing of this data. Informal evaluation should be conducted frequently. The social worker can continuously assess the reactions of employees within the context of informal conversation; listening to the subtle nuances can give a clear picture of how the EAP is really perceived. While formal program assessment is vital for many purposes, the informal assessment often forms a truer picture of the impact of the EAP on the organization.

Clinically, the EAP social worker is concerned about follow-up, continuity of care, and open communication with the referring management/union rep and treatment resources. Peer review can assure the quality of clinical assessment and intervention. All this occurs within the strict policy of confidentiality.

Credibility is crucial to an EAP. The behavior of employees following their contact with the EAP is observable, whether or not others know of the contact. In many ways the EAP assessment is conducted by all "consumers" involved: the individual client, the manager, union representative, co-workers, the department and the organization as a whole. Professional conduct by the social worker in every interaction will go a long way towards credibility.

CONCLUSION

We have discussed numerous aspects of social work assessment in meeting corporate needs through an Employee Assistance Program. We believe that social workers will continue to make a tremendously valuable contribution to American business. First and foremost, we must continue training social workers in the basic tenets of clinical social work. It would be important to teach student social workers more about the business world so as to familiarize them with the corporate culture, norms and expectations. The task, as we see it for the future, will be for social workers to retain their listening, assessment and interviewing skills, while also becoming fully integrated into the world of small and large business.

REFERENCES

Akabas, S.H., Kurzman, P.A. and Kolben, N.S. (1979). *Labor and Industrial Settings: Sites for Social Work Practice*. New York: Council on Social Work Education.

Akabas, S.H. and Kurzman, P.A. (1982). *Work, Workers and Work Organizations*. NJ: Prentice-Hall.

Burden, D.S. and Goggins, B. (1987). *Boston University Balancing Job and Homelife Study*. Boston: Boston University School of Social Work.

Chestang, L.W. (1982). Work, Personnel Change, and Human Development. In Akabas, S.H. and Kurzman, P.A. *Work, Workers and Work Organizations*. NJ: Prentice-Hall, pp. 61-89.

Cohen and McGowan. (1982). What Do You Do? An Inquiry into the Potential Work Related Research. In S.H. Akabas and P.A. Kurzman. *Work, Workers and Work Organizations*. NJ: Prentice-Hall, pp. 117-146.

Deal, T.E. and Kennedy, A. (1982). *Corporate Cultures*, Boston: Addison-Wesley Publishing Co.

Egdahl, R.H., Walsh, D.C. and Goldbeck, W. (eds.) (1980). *Mental Wellness Programs For Employees*. New York: Springer-Verlag.

Erfurt, J.C. and Foote, A. (1977). *Occupational Employee Assistance Programs for Substance Abuse and Mental Health Problems*. University of Michigan, Ann Arbor, MI: Institute of Labor and Industrial Relations.

Feinstein, B.B. and Brown, E.G. (1982). *The New Partnership: Human Services, Business and Industry*. Cambridge, MA: Schenkman Publishing Co.

Hellan, R. and Tisone, C. (1983). EAPs in Adolescence: Still Learning but Damn Smart! *Alcoholism*, July/August, pp. 28-31.

Kantor, R.M. (1977). *Men and Women of the Corporation*. New York: Basic Books.

Kantor, R.M. (1983). *The Change Masters*. New York: Simon and Schuster.

Klarreich, F. (1985). *The Human Resource Management Handbook: Principles and Practices of Employee Assistance Programs*. New York: Praeger Press.

Manuso, J. (ed.) (1983). *Occupational Clinical Psychology*. New York: Praeger Press.

McCarthy, D.E. "The EAP Consultant," in Danto, E. and McConaghy, R. *Employee Assistance: Program for the Future*. Prentice-Hall. (In Press)

McLean, A. (ed.) (1970). *Mental Health and Work Organizations*. Chicago: Rand McNally & Co.

Morton, J.S. and Blake, R.B. (1982). Principles and Designs for Enhancing Learning, *Training and Development Journal*, Vol. pp. 60-63.

Nahrwold, S.C. (1983). Why Programs Fail. J. Manuso (ed.) *Occupational Clinical Psychology*, New York: Praeger Press, pp. 105-115.

Noland, R.L. (ed.) (1973). *Industrial Mental Health and Employee Counseling*. New York: Behavioral Publications.

Perlman, H.H. (1982). The Client as Worker: A Look at an Overlooked Role. In S.H. Akabas and P.A. Kurzmann, pp. 90-116. *Work, Workers and Work Organizations*. New York: Prentice-Hall.

Rosen, R.H. (1988). *Healthy Companies: How People Can Love Their Work, and Companies Can Respect Their People*. New York: St. Martins Press.

Shein, E.H. (1985). *Organizational Culture and Leadership*. San Francisco: Jossey-Bass Publishers.

Spicer, T., Owen, P. and Levine, D. (1983). *Evaluating Employee Assistance Programs*. Minneapolis: Hazelden Foundation.

Straussner, S.L.A. (1988). "Comparison of In House and Contracted-Out Employee Assistance Programs," *Social Work*, Vol. 33, No. 1.

Tuechter, M. and Utne, J. (1982). Wellness: Addressing the Whole Person, *Training and Development Journal*, Vol. pp. 112-16.

Walsh, D.C. (1982). Employee Assistance Programs. *Milbank Memorial Fund Quarterly/Health and Society*. Vol. 60, No. 3, pp. 492-517.

Wrich, J.T. (1984). *The Employee Assistance Program: An Update for the Eighties*. Minneapolis: Hazelden Foundation.

Social Workers in Union-Based Programs

Daniel Molloy
Lynne Burmeister

SUMMARY. Labor-based social work has grown slowly, but steadily, over the last fifteen years. This paper examines developments and conceptualizations assisting the planning and implementation of social service programs in trade unions. Operational framework, skills attractive to labor, and the extensive service assignment are also treated. The paper concludes by highlighting the emergence of an important forum in labor uniting all its helping enterprises. It is a forum in which social work has a key role.

INTRODUCTION

The employment of social workers in American trade unions, as an identifiable phenomenon, is a recent development. The longest running Member Assistance and Social Service Programs, presently in operation, originated in the mid 1970s. Growth could best be described as steady, careful, and cautious. Even now as the labor-social work connection enters its second decade, it would be hard to list more than 150 social workers attached to trade unions for purposes of providing membership services. An additional 50 social workers might be employed by Central Bodies, Labor Agencies, or serve as labor liaisons to community-based programs.

This paper attempts to trace briefly the groundwork leading up to the establishment of labor-based industrial social work programs. It then discusses the framework in which social work is practiced in

Daniel Molloy, DSW, is Director, Personal Service Unit, National Maritime Union Pension & Welfare Plan. Mailing address: 652 59th Street, Brooklyn, NY 11220. Lynne Burmeister, CSW, is Coordinator, Social Service Department, 1199 National Benefit Plan. Mailing address: 1199 National Benefit Fund, 310 W. 43rd Street, New York, NY 10036.

labor, as well as the social work skills to which trade unions most connect. The roles and functions of social workers in trade unions and the various union-based social service programs are illustrated. The paper concludes with a presentation of an important development in labor, which is solidifying the relationship between labor and all its helping components. Social work has a key role in this forum.

DEVELOPMENT AND FRAMEWORK

While sustained social work activity within trade unions began and developed in the 1970s, some more far-reaching historical antecedents are worth noting. Particularly noteworthy was the pioneering work of Bertha Reynolds at the National Maritime Union in the early 1940s (Reynolds, 1951).

Three themes stand out in Reynolds' work. The first centers around her hypothesis that a helping program in a membership organization is less stigmatized. She felt that clients would be more assertive and comfortable and their workers more responsive when, ultimately, the clients owned the program. Secondly, Reynolds saw all social work intervention as an attempt to help both the person and the system. Just treatment in the system was as important as personal modifications: social change went hand in hand with personal change. This was, of course, a perspective trade unions shared. Third, Reynolds believed that social work needed to be provided at the "crossroads of life," closer to the style and substance of everyday living and working. The three critical insights of Reynolds—worker ownership, the social justice theme and social work that is close to social living—are themes still in evidence in union-based social work services and programs.

Weiner, Akabas and Sommer (1973) carried Reynolds' insights further as they conceptualized linkage and partnership between mental health professionals and the world of work. In industrial settings they saw a unique opportunity for a clinical and systems approach to enrich and strengthen each other. Work itself was valued as a key to mental health, although accommodations in the client and/or the work system might be necessary. Like Reynolds, Weiner saw the workplace as a critical locus for service. Clinicians and community agencies needed to become much more aware of the potential of work-based mechanisms to both prevent and help treat problems. Work organizations, in turn, needed to see how sensitive personnel and flexible systems could be of enormous help to a troubled worker. Since Weiner's pioneering work was primarily under union auspices (Amalgamated Clothing and Textile Workers Union), it influenced and contributed conceptually to a number of the union-based programs developing in New York City in the 1970s and spreading throughout the country.

Akabas and Kurzman provide an historical overview on the relationship between social work and work, workers, trade unions, and employers (Akabas and Kurzman, 1982). They describe an ebb and flow in the relationship, times of positive interconnection, partings of the ways, as well as periods of antagonism, suspicion, and mistrust. From their analysis two themes can be extracted to explain the renewed linkage between social work and trade unions during the 1970s.

First, labor and social work seem to grow closer to each other in times of economic crisis. While the national recession in the 1970s ended for many sectors of the economy during the prosperity of the 1980s, it continued unabated in certain older industrial constellations. In such situations when social work looks at social change as well as individual intervention, it is a natural ally with labor. The first theme suggests a second, which is much more far-reaching. Akabas and Kurzman hypothesize that the greater the unity of purpose of labor unions and employing organizations, the more likely the development of a social work role in an industrial setting.

The consequences of these dynamics were twofold: Social work programs have developed in depressed industries, either under labor or joint labor-management auspices. These programs have targeted those most affected by the decline and the erosion taking place in a particular industry. Even more significantly, though, from the perspective of the development of industrial social work in trade unions, was the achievement of consensus in certain labor-management circles that the interests of both were served by meeting the human needs of labor force participants. The achievement of this consensus has taken place in depressed, as well as flourishing, industries. Akabas and Kurzman suggest such consensus came about after more basic wage and fringe benefit goals were obtained and was abetted by progressive occupational legislation of the 1970s — OSHA, EEO, and affirmative action. Perhaps the best expression of the consensus was promoted by the AFL-CIO in its conceptualization of the human contract:

> The human contract, developed by labor and management around the conference table in a climate of cooperation, should concern itself with those personal and family problems which are not covered by the union contract . . . professionals, equipped with a special expertise, can help both management and labor . . . focus attention on the needs of the individual. . . . What every joint union-management committee needs (in every department, on every shift, depending on the number of employees involved) is a professional trained in industrial social work. (Perlis, 1977)

Another important antecedent and link between labor and social work was the concern of both for strong, efficient and quality community-based agencies. The Community Service Department of the AFL-CIO, on both national and state levels, has always considered the strengthening of local programming in the community, as well as gaining full access to such programs for working people, as major goals. Social workers both administer and provide direct service in such agencies. In many communities, labor and community-based social workers have had a working relationship dating back to the Second World War (Straussner and Phillips, 1988).

During the recession of the 1970s as union members turned to their labor organizations for help with extensive and complex human problems, individual unions and central bodies began to look at their own need to provide more direct services and advocacy for workers in large entitlement and treatment systems. Unions began to see their need to become knowledgeable about community resources, to assess and refer expertly, and to help members negotiate through large systems where they could easily get lost. It seemed natural to forge a partnership with and to employ members of a profession with specialized skills, interests, and concerns in these areas.

THE FUNCTION OF SOCIAL WORKERS
IN A TRADE UNION SETTING

Unions have invested considerable time and effort in building natural helping networks. Thousands of union members have completed peer counselor training programs, which aim at giving participants information and referral resources and skills enabling them to respond to a union brother or sister in need. In addition, elected and appointed union officials have helping responsibilities built into the very fabric of their position in the organization.

Social workers must be careful not to compete with or to try displacing these natural union helpers. To attempt to do so would be disastrous and dysfunctional from every aspect. Collaboration, partnership building, and role definition are critical skills. How professional and natural helpers enrich and reinforce each other has been demonstrated in Molloy's study of the National Maritime Union (Molloy, 1986). Natural helpers come to see themselves as the "scouts" within the formal social service network.

Organizational helpers, union officials, tend to see the social worker as a clarifier of issues. The union official wants to understand the individual's or group's need: What is the frequency of the need; how deep are the tensions it is causing? How can the organization respond to it? He needs the social worker to help him understand it, both quickly and in depth.

A social worker in a trade union must be willing and able to work within the existing union framework. Even more, he/she must see it as opportunity, rather than limitation. The social worker can be the beneficiary of the natural helpers referring to the program and providing information about it to the union membership. At the same time, the social worker needs to develop a trusted consultative relationship with union leaders. A social service program not moving in both these directions within a trade union structure risks missed opportunity and sure alienation.

Point of Intervention

A significant portion of the population trade unions represent come from working class background. Income varies enormously, from substantial to near poverty level. Work can be seasonal, putting further stress on income management. Problems almost always have financial issues attached to them. Fear of losing financial insulation and falling into poverty is a preoccupation for many workers; it is an obsession for some and a reality for others.

Social workers in trade unions must take this fear seriously. Responses to psychosocial needs must be orchestrated around addressing financial difficulties.

If a client comes in with enormous medical bills for a spouse, the fiscal problems must be addressed before there can be any meaningful work done on the impact of the illness on the family. Chronic unemployment will require income maintenance assistance woven carefully around treating a client's depression.

It could, and should, be maintained that this is good social work practice in any setting. However, the mixture of concrete and clinical services is a centerpiece in most trade union settings. In almost every intervention, a social worker will need to engage his/her client on a level of basic human needs, in addition to intrapsychic and interpersonal assessment and treatment.

Traditional Social Work Skills
Attractive to Labor

Some traditional social work skills are particularly attractive to trade unions. First, unions and their benefit plans are themselves complex organizations, existing in an even more complex environment. Social work skills and values are woven around people, as well as social systems. A union member needs help in utilizing his/her occupational benefit system and if necessary, a public entitlement system, as efficiently and effectively as possible. The best possible accommodations between the available resources and the member's needs must be arranged. The social worker tries to master systems and help clients navigate through them.

Secondly, social workers frequently combine clinical and administrative skills, allowing them to move from identifying needs to developing programs. As social workers begin to understand, document, and attempt addressing individual needs, themes emerge. The themes suggest where the needs originate, as well as the personal and organizational resources which may be available to address them. The programs can be targeted at a specific population as described below. Programs are conceptualized, planned, implemented, and ultimately evaluated. Program building skills, while not unique to social work, are an integral part of the profession's expertise.

Finally, social workers' orientation, values and methods are close to labor's own principles and concerns. The casework model takes an almost casuistic approach, cataloging the ingenious solutions clients find to difficult problems. It is more concerned with strength than pathology. Finding, analyzing, supporting, and operationalizing personal and organizational strengths is a skill particularly important to working people, who may be in difficulty, but who still have relatively intact lives. Labor is always looking to activate individual member and collective strengths and is comfortable with professional skills which systematically attempt to meet need with strengths.

SOCIAL SERVICE PROGRAMS IN UNIONS

Social service programs in unions are usually housed in the union's Health and Welfare Fund or Pension and Welfare Plan. They may be totally discrete entities within the Fund or be associated with a Health Unit. In most cases, social service programs report directly to a Plan or Fund Administrator. However, there are almost always formal and informal mechanisms for operational consultation from the union itself.

Social service programs in unions are in many cases a labor-management benefit. Arrived through a labor-management agreement and supported by both, the union has usually been the primary protagonist in the pursuit of the program or has maintained that such programs are worthwhile allocations of limited benefit dollars.

Unions have tended to look to their social service programs in addressing targeted needs in five general areas:

1. Mental Health
2. Chemical Dependency
3. Family Issues (e.g., daycare, single parenting pressures, family dysfunction)

4. Entitlements
5. Consultation with labor and management whenever any of the above impact on work itself.

Provision of union-based services is usually offered within an assessment-referral-aftercare model, with brief and even long-term treatment available in some circumstances.

All of these issues cannot be covered within the scope of this paper and some are not unlike service provision in settings other than labor. Some services provided are similar to those offered by an EAP. What is unique to labor is the extensive population which is its constituency. To demonstrate this, the paper describes the four targeted groups labor is attending to particularly at this time, and how social workers are involved in the provision of service. It might be said that social service programs in unions are Member Assistance Programs at their base plus much more. The "much more" is the potential program planning and development around a problem or constituency to which labor feels responsible and for which both labor and social work feel social service has a role to play in the helping process.

TARGETED GROUPS FOR SERVICE

Retirees

As our population ages, so does the population within labor unions. This coupled with the decline in union membership due to the shift from a manufacturing to a service economy, makes the retired segment of unions much more prominent. This group is generally composed of members who may have helped form their respective unions and thus are experienced in speaking out and standing up for their rights.

Retirees generally face many challenges which converge at a time of life when energy and supports may have diminished considerably. Their concerns have to do with such fundamental needs as medical care and income, as well as changed self-images and other intangible issues. Programs and resources become highly necessary at this time to help preserve and maintain the quality of life for these individuals. Labor unions and their social workers provide tremendous support and help to this needy group.

The health status of retirees is variable as advances in medical care have prolonged life. Individuals may suffer from physical diseases, or they may find themselves physically sound but mentally debilitated.

Unions, in conjunction with physicians and medical facilities, have developed programs which assess and treat individuals for a variety of medical problems ranging from cardiovascular health to breast cancer. Such assessment programs not only can improve the lives of retired workers; they can also detect developing health problems among younger workers so that their health status upon retiring is improved.

Union-based social workers work collaboratively with these health assessment programs to provide supportive counseling to members first learning that their health is impaired. Such counseling can enable individuals to grieve over the loss of "perfect" health and help them to adjust to changes in routines that can improve or preserve their health status. Additionally, social workers work with individuals who are noncompliant with treatment regimens and help them work through their resistance to making needed changes in their routines.

Most labor unions which have pension funds in turn have staff who monitor these funds and the benefits provided to their retirees.

Seminars and materials are generally provided to educate and prepare new and prospective retirees for the transition. Preretirement seminars are a mainstay of these programs and the vehicle through which this information is disseminated. Frequently social workers are called upon to explain services and agencies in the community that work strictly with retired individuals or those 60 years of age and above. Such information regarding available programs paves the way for retired individuals to link up with new outlets for socialization as well as with financial and other services that can ease the restrictions imposed by fixed incomes.

Another component of preretirement programs focuses on the psychological adjustment that must take place in order for retirees to move smoothly into retirement. Social workers frequently apply the psychosocial model of Erik Erikson (1959) with regard to retirees, and understand that by allowing individuals to discuss and examine their changes in perspective and role status, they can better master the skills that this new phase of life requires. Social workers also possess knowledge of crisis theory and how changes and stressors in life can bring about a crisis. Intervention through individual and group counseling or discussion can enable individuals to achieve a level of growth through the period of crisis that retirement often precipitates.

Finally, community organizing skills are crucial in helping union retirees. Such knowledge base can enable social workers to set up, or provide technical assistance in setting up, activities and community groups of retirees. These activities not only provide companionship; they also structure the day and can help reticent retirees develop their leadership skills. Retirees clubs or associations allow retirees to maintain their relationships with former co-workers as well as to develop new friendships with people in their community who also happen to be retired from the same union. Such programs have become an integral component of many pension and retirement programs within unions.

The energy exhibited by many retirees, as well as their increased free time, has made them a perfect group to tap for assistance to other union members in need. Various labor unions have developed programs staffed by volunteer retirees under the supervision of social workers who reach out to homebound retirees or disabled working members. These programs have proven to be highly effective in making retirees feel needed as well as in reaching a population which would not otherwise receive services.

Disabled Workers

Having to leave work temporarily or permanently due to a disabling medical condition is a fear that all too often becomes a reality for many workers. It doesn't matter if the injury or illness occurred on or off the job. The most prominent loss is likely to be the reduction or discontinuation of income. Disability payments through union benefit funds or state disability funds represent only a portion of worker's salaries. Workers who are injured on the job may receive workers compensation payments which also amount to only a portion of regular salary. In some cases they may receive only partial payments or payments to cover medical expenses. Cases that are controverted, not accepted by the worker's Compensation Board, may render individuals ineligible for payments. These cases may then require hearing after hearing and continued submission of medical evidence pertaining to the injury.

When workers have exhausted their disability benefits and their disabling condition remains, they may need to apply for Social Security Disability benefits. This process is generally unfamiliar, threatening and arduous for most workers. Individuals may be turned down for benefits or may have to appeal the declination, perhaps several times. Thus, workers need somewhere to turn to obtain help and an understanding of these programs. Social workers can prove invaluable throughout these processes.

Knowledge of the application processes, as well as, the eligibility criteria for union disability programs, Worker's Compensation and Social Security Disability are crucial for social workers working with union members. Supportive counseling as well as advocacy can prove invaluable in guiding disabled members through the maze of bureaucracy.

In some cases, social workers may be able to expedite decisions for eligibility as well as acquisition of benefits.

The financial strain imposed by reduced income often puts workers in the position where they need to apply for public assistance, food stamps and Medicaid. These systems can at the same time overwhelm those who need to use them. Social workers can provide counseling, guidance and advocacy to assist workers with this process. They can be particularly helpful with workers who feel shamed by the need to secure entitlements.

Dislocated Workers

Labor unions have felt the brunt of the shift in the U.S. economy seen during the past two decades as service industries have replaced manufacturing as the predominant mode of employment. These sweeping economic changes have forced labor unions to provide help to their memberships in adjusting to layoffs and dislocation. Social workers provide assistance with stress management, and the psychosocial ramifications of job loss, as well as information regarding unemployment insurance benefit programs and job service programs. Many labor unions have set up meetings for dislocated members with representatives from these Department of Labor programs in order to assist their members with the application process for unemployment insurance benefits and enrollment with job service. Social workers who are familiar with these programs and the special provisions available to specific groups of dislocated workers can insure that these workers are getting all to which they are entitled.

Because shop and plant closings have become so commonplace, states offices of the AFL-CIO can be extremely effective in securing monies to establish comprehensive programs for dislocated workers. In New York State, the state office of the AFL-CIO establishes Worker Assistance/Re-employment Centers to assist large numbers of dislocated workers. These centers utilize union resources such as social service departments in addition to city and state training and entitlement programs.

Labor unions whose members are experiencing shop and plant closings may also be approached by city agencies such as Departments of Education with contracts to provide job development and direct job placement opportunities. Members are screened and linked up with jobs that best match their skills and abilities. While this process appears simple, it is rife with obstacles. Workers whose skills lie in certain areas may have trouble finding an occupation to which their skills will transfer. Social workers within labor unions can act as liaisons between these programs and workers. Barriers to utilization of these programs such as literacy or child care needs can be addressed by social workers through referrals to necessary programs or services.

Legal Services Programs

Labor unions, specifically, and the AFL-CIO as a whole, have recognized that union members often find legal assistance to be financially prohibitive. To counter this obstacle, the Union Privilege Legal Services Program was developed for AFL-CIO members and their families.

Attorneys were chosen for this program based on their sensitivity to labor unions as well as their willingness to offer reduced rates for services. Union members can receive free consultations, free document review, and certain free follow-up services. Social workers assist members with the referral process and provide assistance with non-legal matters such as securing marriage counseling or alternative housing options.

Many local unions choose to develop their own legal programs. Some function in-house with a hired staff of attorneys who work closely with social workers. Often the social workers will conduct intake interviews to determine the nature of the problem, whether legal or otherwise.

Other legal programs organize panels of attorneys which members can utilize or arrange for firms to provide "legal nights" during which members can obtain legal consultation. In these settings, social workers work collaboratively with the attorneys to resolve the non-legal aspects of their legal problems.

PRESENT DEVELOPMENTS

Experience has shown that the development of social service departments within labor unions has proved to be invaluable to members in many facets of their lives.

While labor is increasingly engaging social workers, it is doing so with balance, caution, and purpose. Given labor's commitment to respond to a variety of personal, social, educational, health, and legal needs, no single profession will ever enjoy labor's exclusive patronage. Labor also continues to support and cultivate natural helpers and its peer counseling training programs. There is a sense that a union member serving a union member is not only necessary for a full extension of helping programs but is also in many cases the most appropriate form of intervention. Along these lines there is a growing sense that a partnership needs to develop among labor leaders responsible for human service provision, trained peer counselors and natural helpers, and the professional helpers. They all have a role to play in planning, implementing and delivering human services within trade unions. Their various perspectives complement and enrich each other.

This partnership can be illustrated by the success and growth of the Human Service Providers Advisory Committee (HSPAC) within the labor community in New York City. HSPAC is an advisory committee on human services to the New York City Central Labor Council. It includes an Executive Board, Sub-Committees and rests on the foundation of a Network. The goal of the Network is to provide a forum for all "labor-based human service providers under the umbrella of the New York City Central Labor Council, AFL-CIO, to share information and resources and to exchange views." The Community Service Departments of the National AFL-CIO and the New York State Federation of the AFL-CIO, labor-based social workers, other labor-based human service providers, and the New York City Central Labor Rehabilitation Council all saw the need for such a forum and played a critical part in its development.

The importance of this Committee can but be appreciated by a listing of its objectives (HSPAC, 1988):

1. Promote the ideals, values, and objectives of the labor movement through the activities of human services providers at the Central Labor Council.
2. Provide a central resource center to serve the human service program needs of labor human service providers so that they may better meet the needs and aspirations of workers, their families, and retirees.
3. Inform the public about the services provided to workers and retirees by unions through their human services employees and volunteers.
4. Advise concerned organizations and individuals about the quality, quantity, and variety of service delivery methods of labor organizations.
5. Effectively collaborate with local, regional, and national governmental and voluntary human service organizations on the human service needs of working people and the accessibility of services.
6. Collect and disseminate appropriate data, conduct surveys and research projects to improve and extend the body of knowledge concerning human services.
7. Study new service delivery approaches and address new issues

of concern to workers as outlined in the AFL-CIO's report on "The Changing Situation of Workers and Their Unions."

8. Provide opportunities for labor human service workers to strengthen their skills; to strengthen and unify their commitment to the labor movement as a locus for human services.

CONCLUSION

Labor has substantially expanded the base of its human service provision in an increasingly complex world. In doing so it has held on to its long tradition of the peer helper and counselor, while forging partnerships with professionals to develop discrete program entities to address special and complex needs. The challenge now is to unite all these efforts, so that they are mutually supportive, increasingly effective, and are in line with the best traditions and values of both labor and social work.

REFERENCES

Akabas, Sheila and Paul Kurzman. (Eds.) (1982). *Work, Workers and Work Organizations.* Englewood Cliffs, NJ: Prentice Hall.

Erikson, Erik. (1959). *Identity and the Life Cycle*, Psychological Issues, I. New York: International Universities Press.

Molloy, Daniel. (1986). *Planning and Implementing a Worker-Based and Participating Model for Employee Assistance Programs.* New York: Graduate Center, CUNY, Doctoral Dissertation.

Parad, Howard J. (ed.) (1965). *Crisis Intervention: Selected Readings.* New York: Family Service Association of America.

Perlis, Leo. (Winter, 1977). "The Human Contract in the Organized Workplace." *Social Thought*, No. 1, 29-35.

Reynolds, Bertha. (1951). *Social Work and Social Living.* Washington, DC: NASW Classics.

Sonnenstuhl, William and Harrison Trice. (1986). *Strategies for Employee Assistance Programs: The Crucial Balance.* New York: Cornell University, New York School of Industrial and Labor Relations.

Straussner, Shulamith, L. A. and Norma Phillips. (March, 1988). Social Work and Labor Unions. *Journal of Sociology and Social Welfare*: Vol XV, No. 1.

Trice, Harrison and Paul Roman. (1978). *Spirits and Demons at Work: Alcohol and Drugs on the Job.* New York: Cornell University, New York State School of Industrial and Labor Relations.

Weiner, Hyman, Sheila Akabas and John Sommer. (1973). *Mental Health in the World of Work.* New York: Association Press.

Managed Mental Health Care for Employees: Roles for Social Workers

Jacqueline Bloom Wagman
Jeanette Schiff

SUMMARY. Managed mental health care has become an increasingly significant influence in the timely, appropriate and cost-conscious delivery of mental health and substance abuse services. Social workers are being presented with new career paths in the private sector as EAP programs and managed health care corporations look to them to provide the case review, supervision, provider selection, and the quality assurance functions of a well integrated managed health care system.

Managed Mental Health Care came into existence as a response to escalating costs associated with treatment and the rapidly increasing health benefit premiums. This is reflected in the costs of the "total health care insurance premiums which rose from $25 billion in 1973 to $11 billion in 1983, a four fold increase while the employer's share of private health insurance premiums has increased at an average annual rate of 16% during the same ten year period" (Yadrick & Rothermel, 1988: 15). This article discusses the rise of health care costs, particularly for mental health and chemical dependency and the development of managed mental health care sys-

Jacqueline Bloom Wagman, CSW, CEAP, is Director, Employee Assistance Program Development, Preferred Health Care, Ltd. Jeanette Schiff, ACSW, is Director, Network Development, Preferred Health Care, Ltd. Address correspondence to the authors at Preferred Health Care Ltd., 15 River Rd. Suite 300, Wilton Center, Wilton, CT 06897.

tems in the 1980s. The article also discusses the roles of social workers within the evolving managed mental health system.

DEVELOPMENT OF MANAGED MENTAL HEALTH CARE

Prior to the uncontrollable inflation of the late 1970s and early 1980s, employees had come to expect health benefits as a requisite benefit of their employment. Employers at that time were not cost-conscious purchasers of mental health care since psychiatric and substance abuse treatment was a relatively small part of the total health care bill. Insurance carriers also did not experience benefi-ciaries extensively utilizing their benefits and therefore were disin-clined to trim the cost of these services. Their role was simply that of providing a vehicle for handling the payment of health care ren-dered by bona fide providers. Few benefit options were provided and the employer simply purchased whatever the carriers offered in regards to mental health plans.

However, during the 1970s health and mental health care premi-ums and costs began to rise due to a number of factors including:

- Oversupply of hospital beds.
- Oversupply of physicians and an increased number of mental health providers eligible for third party reimbursement.
- Commercialization/overbuilding/advertising of psychiatric and chemical dependency hospitals.
- Reduction in the stigmatization of those seeking psychiatric treatment. This resulted in heightened social responsibility among employers to offer professional counseling for personal and family problems in health benefit plans.
- Expanded use of benefits for substance abuse and mental health problems.
- Limited experience of traditional plan administrators with psy-chiatric benefits cost design and terminology.

Payors of health benefits became alarmed by requests for reim-bursement of services that were lengthy and expensive. As a re-sponse to these rising costs employers and insurance carriers imple-mented health plans that had high deductibles, co-payments, and out-of-pocket expenses. However these plans did not contain the continual escalation of costs. The purchasers of health benefits began asking "how do we control costs?" and "are all of these treatments really medically necessary?"

To answer these questions, Utilization Review Programs (UR) were developed. These consisted of paper-based, retrospective reviews of diagnosis and length of stay. The purpose was to curtail benefit payment for long-term or medically unnecessary treatment for medical/surgical patients. The reviews were primarily conducted by nurses with medical/surgical backgrounds who were employed by major insurance companies. While UR programs were reducing hospitals' lengths of stay, they were not saving money within the total continuum of care. Claims for outpatient services rose as diagnoses were changed by providers when the limits of reimbursement under one part of the health care plan were exhausted.

Moreover, the often cumbersome and inefficient method of retrospective review of psychiatric and substance abuse treatment had been shown to be generally burdensome on mental health professionals and treatment facilities. Financial hardships for patients and providers alike ensued from retrospective denials. In addition many payors have found the cost of operating large utilization review programs prohibitive, as well as generally ineffective, in influencing the quality of care provided to their beneficiaries.

As a result employers began to consider capping, limiting and cutting health benefits at a time when "the demand for mental health services and substance abuse services has continued to increase" (Rodriguez & Macher, 1986: 14). The result was the emergence of managed mental health care systems.

DEFINITION OF MANAGED MENTAL HEALTH CARE

Managed Mental Health Care can briefly be described as the development and implementation of a mental health benefit plan that controls costs while assuring that the quality of care being delivered is not sacrificed. The key components of a managed mental health care plan are the following:

- Confidential assessment and triage
- Pre-certification and pre-admission review
- Concurrent clinical case review
- Discharge planning with linkage to alternative levels of care
- A selected provider panel of individual practitioners, programs and facilities
- Integrated claims processing system
- Built-in financial incentives which may include:
  - higher level of benefit payment
  - reduced or waived co-payment
  - no out-of-pocket expenses to the beneficiary
  - increased annual or lifetime benefits

The unique aspect of a managed mental health care plan as opposed to the retrospective utilization review plan, is the concurrent clinical review. Typically, these reviewers are licensed and experienced clinical professionals from the major mental health disciplines of Social Work, Psychology, Psychiatry, and Nursing. Their role is the ongoing review of treatment that is being delivered by the providers and the authorization of benefit payments. It is in this capacity that social workers have found a new career avenue into the corporate world.

THE ASSESSMENT AND REFERRAL/
PRE-CERTIFICATION STAGE

The main social work skills on which managed care is premised and functions from are assessment and referral. The psychosocial assessment and determining a DSM III diagnosis begins the treatment process. By assessing the individual's level of functioning, their strengths and weakness, and the social/occupational and familial pressures that the individual is responding to, an opinion about the overall dysfunction is established.

Once these factors are explored and the clinical picture becomes clearer, the managed care clinician forms a probable diagnosis and refers the individual into an appropriate level of treatment with a provider whose assessment and ongoing treatment will either confirm or contradict the original diagnosis. The initial assessment and diagnosis determines the necessity and the initial length of psychiatric treatment which is then pre-certified or authorized by the clinical case manager. The pre-admission review will involve contact with the patient and/or type of facility and level of intensity of treatment suited to the individual patient needs.

After the initial assessment by a clinical case manager is completed, a referral to a provider who specializes in the identified problem area(s) is made. The referral sets the direction for the treatment, and throughout the treatment process the managed care clinical case manager determines the appropriateness of care which is offered/provided and authorizes benefit payment.

CLINICAL CONCURRENT REVIEW STAGE

The goals and objectives of the treatment plans usually change as the patient improves and needs different level of care. Clinical concurrent case review is the process of reviewing such treatment goals and determining benefit payments as each new phase of treatment emerges.

Concurrent clinical case review necessitates periodic contact with the patient and provider to assure the continued appropriateness and the medical necessity of treatment. The role of the clinical case manager during the referral/concurrent clinical case review stage adds an extra layer of support to the patient's treatment since the reviewer also functions as a patient advocate with the provider to assure proper treatment.

The criteria utilized to insure that the level of treatment and care is appropriate to the individual needs of the patient are based on a variety of national and state guidelines such as the American Academy of Child and Adolescent Psychiatry, American Psychiatric Association, Civilian Health and Medical Program of the Uniformed Services, State Divisions of Alcoholism, and so on.

EMPLOYEE ASSISTANCE PROGRAMS AND MANAGED MENTAL HEALTH CARE

Employee Assistance Programs (EAPs), as an important component of human service departments of most major employers, are increasingly playing a central role in the management of mental health and chemical dependency benefits (Lightman & Wagman, 1988). EAPs have developed distinct managed mental health care systems which complement and formalize their traditional role. A core component for many managed mental health care systems is the heavy involvement of EAPs in benefit coordination as the gatekeeper of treatment. The following models describe the components in which an EAP plays a significant role in managing the mental health care for employees.

Model 1

This model has been implemented for use with both internal and external EAPs. In this model the EAP has no direct control over payment, but consults with and advises the insurance carrier. The components of this model are as follows:

1. The EAP fulfills the assessment and gatekeeper functions.
2. The employee is educated about the benefit options and financial incentives of EAP utilization. The education is provided jointly by the company and EAP. The financial incentives may include:

   • reduced or waived copayments.
   • higher benefit reimbursement payment.
   • payment to provider directly from insurance carrier.
   • no claim forms.
   • approval for alternate providers who are not traditionally covered by an insurance carrier, e.g., clinical social workers.

3. Treatment programs and facilities may also re-route self-referred employees to the EAP to benefit from the aforementioned financial incentives.
4. The EAP develops a formal Preferred Provider (PPO) contractual arrangement with treatment facilities and programs.
5. The insurance carrier contracts with the approved facilities as a PPO.
6. The EAP sends a letter of pre-certification to the facility to authorize treatment.

7. The facility submits the EAP pre-certification letter to the insurance carrier with the bill.
8. The EAP monitors treatment/concurrent clinical case review/discharge planning. Lines of communication run between the EAP and treatment provider, as well as the provider and insurance carrier.
9. The EAP follows up with the employee to verify that the services have been obtained and the procedures followed. Also, the EAP follows up with the insurance carrier to approve treatment and payment of mental health benefits, or if necessary the EAP consults with the provider and insurance carrier on alternative treatment recommendations.

Model 2

This model was designed for the internal EAP which has direct control over the benefit payment. In this model the EAP has the authority, along with the medical director, to stop payment for inappropriate care, much as in the traditional function of an insurance carrier. This model functions as follows:

1. The EAP fulfills the assessment and gatekeeper functions.
2. No employee is reimbursed for any treatment without utilizing the EAP service.
3. The EAP develops a formal PPO arrangement with treatment facilities/programs.
4. The EAP has complete access to insurance claims for employees requesting treatment. This information is used to clarify the employee's psychiatric or substance abuse treatment history.
5. Treatment programs must contact the EAP in order to assure coverage and to verify the worker's eligibility to use benefits.
6. The EAP verifies the eligibility of the worker.
7. The EAP sends a letter of pre-certification to the facility to authorize treatment.
8. The facility must submit information to the EAP regarding the admitting symptoms, tentative diagnosis, treatment plan, and the expected length of stay.
9. The EAP reviews all insurance claims and authorizes pay-

ment through the work organization's insurance claims office.
10. Payment is made directly to the treatment program via the insurance claims office.
11. The EAP monitors treatment/concurrent review/discharge planning. The provider sends UR materials to the EAP.
12. The EAP consults with the provider on alternative treatment recommendations, if necessary.
13. The EAP follows up with the employee to verify that the services have been obtained and the procedures followed.

SOCIAL WORK AND MANAGED CARE

Clinical social work has evolved in public and private agencies which emphasized the counselling and psychotherapeutic skills of their professional staff. Mental health settings, in particular, have employed social workers to provide individual, group and family therapy across the continuum from intensive inpatient facilities to numerous outpatient programs and clinics. As the profession has gained in status and recognition as a legitimate provider of mental health services, opportunities for practice have emerged in the private sector. The emergence of managed mental health care and EAPs has added yet another area of practice to the increasing array of employment opportunities for the modern-day social worker.

Within the managed mental health care field, social workers function as clinical case managers, as senior case managers, as evaluators of provider networks, and as developers of policies and programs. A discussion of their roles is provided below.

THE CLINICAL CASE MANAGER

The clinical case manager or reviewer is the backbone of the managed health care process. The case manager provides the interface between health care providers, the client, and the third party payor designated to underwrite the cost of care.

It is this clinician who handles initial requests for referral to a treatment provider at an appropriate level of care. Often this frontline individual responds to crisis situations and is analogous to the intake worker or the crisis-line professional within a social agency. Subsequent to the initial referral the clinical case reviewer maintains an ongoing dialogue with the treatment provider to assure the timely and appropriate delivery of care and the provision of a less intense level of treatment as soon as clinically feasible. The process of triage and case review requires knowledge of psychotherapeutic techniques, variety of treatment modalities and knowledge of treatment resources and of the wide array of health care delivery systems. The skill of interacting comfortably as a case reviewer with other professionals at all levels of competence is another important facet of the case manager. The social worker is in an ideal position to provide the peer consultation that the case review process in a managed health care environment requires.

Clinical acumen for the social worker expands because of the opportunity to interact with colleagues in numerous settings across a wide geographic expanse. A sensitivity to regional and cultural differences becomes an important aspect of the clinical discussions that social work with its attention to social environment is especially adept at. These professional collaborations enlarge the horizons of the case manager from the usual narrow field of the local provider community to a regional and often national level.

The following case describes the clinical process within a managed mental health care system and the role of the case manager:

Sue, a 44-year-old married woman and mother of two adolescent children agreed to seek psychiatric help after two months of increasing feelings of hopelessness, sadness and worthlessness. Her ability to function at a general clerical job had declined significantly in recent weeks and her consumption of alcohol had escalated to several glasses of hard liquor nightly. She had begun to express persistent suicidal ideation with references to the futility of continuing her life and the wish that her struggle could be over. Her husband was supportive but relatively unaware of her emotional stress. She called the health benefits triage line which is on contract with her employer and provided by her insurance carrier. She had a brief discussion with the hot-line clinician assigned to handle psychiatric and substance abuse referrals. Based on this phone call it was recommended that she seek a consultation that day. With her approval, she was referred to a psychiatrist because the clinical picture raised the significant possibility that hospitalization was necessary.

In consultation with Sue and the psychiatrist, the clinician determined that she was in need of inpatient psychiatric treatment. After a two week hospitalization at a psychiatric facility, the attending psychiatrist and the case manager, who was monitoring the treatment on behalf of the health plan, concurred that her symptoms had abated and she no longer needed the intensity of treatment and protection that the hospital had provided. However, she continued to be mildly depressed and unable to resume all of her daily functions, including return to work.

The case manager and the psychiatrist agreed that a period of further intensive treatment could appropriately be provided in a partial hospital setting where she could be involved in specific therapeutic activities for six hours daily and her family could attend an ancillary support group. After five weeks of this program the case reviewer and the partial hospital staff agreed that Sue was able to begin a gradual return to work and the psychiatrist decided to gradually discharge her from the program. Sue elected to continue individual therapy with a social worker who was one of the practitioners suggested to her from a panel of private therapists that the case reviewer and treatment program had determined met her therapeutic needs and were geographically accessible to her. The individual therapy was reviewed monthly until both the case manager and the therapist agreed that Sue's depression had remitted, the substance abuse was no longer an issue, and Sue was functioning well both at home and on the job.

In the above case the reviewer played several significant roles. First of all, during the initial assessment and triage the reviewer had to evaluate the acuity of the patient's symptoms and make a determination about the urgency and the probable level of care indicated. Thereafter, contact had to be maintained with the treatment team through regular treatment reviews in order to assure that the patient had access to a less restrictive level of care when her mental status would permit. This allowed the patient to experience the least amount of disruption to her life and to return to home, family, and work as soon as possible. It thereby also saved her insurance carrier the added expense of a prolonged hospitalization by offering an intermediate level of care as soon as clinically appropriate.

SENIOR CLINICAL CASE MANAGERS

A second employment opportunity for the clinical social worker exists at the supervisory level where senior and experienced managed health care clinicians have a role analogous to that of the traditional agency supervisor. Typically, all supervisory skills are linked to the knowledge of direct practice as well as the ability to comfortably oversee and direct the work of others. Case reviews are monitored by senior staff who provide the supervision and consultation to a group of case managers responsible for a specific region, group of corporate accounts, or specific level of care. Because of the existence of a supervisory structure, professional growth is enhanced and the opportunity of a career ladder within the corporate structure is available.

For both the clinical case manager and the senior case manager a clear understanding of the various mental disorders, the traditional treatment methodologies and innovative treatment approaches is clearly required. Hands-on experience in the provision of care at various settings and the ability to discern the medically/psychologically necessary level and duration of care is equally important.

REVIEWERS OF PROVIDER NETWORKS

The opportunities for social workers do not end with the case management department. A truly comprehensive managed mental health care environment presumes the identification of well-qualified and well managed psychiatric and substance abuse programs and treatment providers. This identification process demands a clinical review of the programs, be they inpatient or outpatient, through on-site discussions and a detailed analysis of their strengths as well as weakness. This process, a separate function from the case review process, is clearly a highly sophisticated activity that demands an awareness not only of the key clinical factors involved in the delivery of good mental health and substance abuse services but also of issues around utilization review and quality assurance. Knowledge of organizational and program design as well as staffing patterns are especially important. The program reviewer must be able to delve into the area of mental health administration while using practice wisdom in the assessment process. This is an exciting arena of applied clinical skills in that it provides the social worker with the chance to survey and assess the complete array of direct services across a wide geographic expanse.

Treatment provider networks are composed of institutional programs and outpatient mental health and substance abuse treatment professionals. They are identified, selected and organized into a provider network after undergoing a review process. The review process screens provider qualifications against national standards for program structures, practitioner credentials, as well as criteria and indicators of quality, utilization efficiency and performance.

POLICY, PROCEDURES
AND PROGRAM DEVELOPERS

Although relatively few in number, some social workers are finding themselves involved in the corporate role of setting standards of policy and procedures within managed mental health care both for the case management review process as well as the development of provider networks.

Developing a successful managed mental health care plan requires the implementation of a case management system with overall emphasis on the following:

1. Development of standardized policies regarding case management.
2. Determining clinical criteria for admission and length of stay at all levels of care.

3. Development of company employee educational programs describing managed mental health care services. Educational programs and materials may include: brochures, letters, employee and supervisory orientation.
4. Provision of case management staff training focusing on assessment, cost-containment, clinical skill development, pharmacology and problem resolution.
5. Monitoring the case management system through quality assurance guidelines and activities.

CONCLUSION

While in its infancy, managed mental health care has presented social workers with a serendipitous career opportunity rather than a career ladder. As the field becomes more mature, it will develop as an avenue for the clinician who is competent to blend direct practice with administrative expertise. It is another avenue for those social workers who are seeking new ways to apply previously learned clinical, administrative, and organizational skills.

As the field of managed mental health care grows, additional education and training in health care administration will be required as the need for that area of knowledge becomes more clearly defined. Social Work education will need to address the emerging role of managed mental health care and incorporate into clinical practicums the exposure to this alternative mental health delivery system.

REFERENCES

Burda, David (July 15, 1988) "Borrowing the Quality Model." *Modern Health Care*, PP 24-32.

Hollis, Florence (1972) *Casework: A Psychosocial Therapy*. New York: Random House.

Kadushin, Alfred (1976) *Supervision in Social Work*. New York: Columbia University Press.

Lightman, Robin & Wagman, Jacqueline (May, 1988). "A Working Proposal for EAPs." *Almacan*, PP 18-21 May Issue.

Mahoney, John, MD, MPH. (May, 1987) "EAP's and Medical Cost Containment." *Almacan*, PP 16-20.

Montgomery, Robert H. (May, 1987) "Alcoholism Treatment Benefits?" *Almacan*, PP 22-25.

Ruffenach, Glenn (Dec. 20, 1988) "Health Costs." *The Wall Street Journal*.

Shalowitz, Deborah (Dec. 5, 1988) "Health Care Spending Tops $500 Billion." *Business Insurance*.

Yandrick, Rudy and Rothermel, Scott (May, 1988) "Health Care, Costs on a Collision Course." *Almacan*, PP 15-17.

Application of Social Work Skills to Human Resource Management

Philip A. Berry

SUMMARY. Workers in various settings are beset with a multitude of issues which sometimes interfere with their personal effectiveness and overall productivity. The skills and knowledge that social workers possess can be applied to nontraditional settings in novel ways to increase employee productivity and organizational effectiveness.

This paper will explore how social work skills can enhance the methods that human resource management applies to the current problems of the workplace. It will examine the skills used by social workers and how those skills uniquely fit with the approaches used in human resources.

TODAY'S UNIQUE WORK ENVIRONMENT

Today the world of work is much more unpredictable and unstable than previously. Corporate mergers, foreign competition, consumer demand and the global economy create a situation where change is constant and the pace of business is frenetic. Plant closures, shifts in federal budgetary attention, crime, AIDS, and drug abuse impact on everybody, and create a more frustrating, and at the same time, more challenging work environment. The shifts in the world economy and the U.S. business scene cannot be divided from the other realities that people function in. Moreover the workplace is not immune to the societal ills plaguing the cities.

Previously, problems like drug abuse, alcoholism, and AIDS, were thought to be related to a limited section of our society. Community and not-for-profit organizations sought to solve these prob-

---

Philip A. Berry, MSW, MBA, is Vice President, Human Resources & Administration, Triborough Bridge and Tunnel Authority, Randall's Island, NY 10035.

lems which were thought to be relegated to the public domain. The solutions were viewed as in individual's personal problem, not the responsibility of the employer. We now realize that these problems are not foreign to the corporate suites and the world of work. These problems also have no respect to race, sex or income level.

PROBLEMS FACING TODAY'S WORKER

The employees of today must often overcome a number of obstacles in their personal and family life to be productive on the job. The employee has numerous other roles which contribute to his/her total being, such as parent, spouse, sibling, community volunteer, civic leader, church member, and so on. The increase of leisure time, the eight-hour average work day and the ability of technology to decrease the time devoted to handling mundane household chores, all allow people to get involved in a number of different activities.

Mass transportation and increased modes of communication also allow people to get involved in many more activities than may have been envisioned years ago.

A breakdown in any of these roles can have a profound impact on the ability of an employee to function well in other roles. When children are having problems at school, the worker's attention and emotion may be diverted from his/her job, possibly leading to poor productivity. If an employee is having difficulty getting work goals accomplished, this can lead to tension in the household with his/her spouse. Problems of adjusting in one area can be extremely stressful, making it difficult to cope in other areas. This difficulty manifests itself in increased rates of absenteeism, tardiness, and lower productivity levels. Increased rates of disability claims is another manifestation. For some, alcohol or controlled substances is used to help cope with a seemingly complex situation.

THE CHANGING WORKFORCE:
GENDER AND MULTICULTURAL AWARENESS

Many more women are working now than previously. The number of women staying at home with the kids is diminishing. The high industrialism of our economy has resulted in an expansion of the service sector which has provided many opportunities for women to work.

Consequently many companies and unions have had to develop child care programs, paternity/maternity leave policies, and flex-time. Many organizations have had to reexamine the qualifications and descriptions for certain jobs. How much strength or endurance is really required to be a fireperson, dock worker, railroad engineer or construction person? What assumptions are made about a woman's ability to handle this work?

It is not uncommon to see male secretaries, flight attendants or nurses. More and more "genderless" jobs exist. This has tremendous implications in terms of language and perception. No longer can we assume that the mail carrier is the postman. Policeman, fireman, and even chairman, are no longer appropriate terminology. Another implication of "genderless" jobs is that we can no longer assume that a mechanic, doctor, electrical engineer or astronaut will always be a male.

The stress on men and women as they change to adapt to these conditions can be tremendous. Both men and women need to learn new ways of adapting, perceiving and behaving in the workplace. Social events like after-work socializing, men's clubs and sports events, need to be examined to insure inclusiveness and not exclusiveness.

Hispanics, African-Americans and Asians are also more of a permanent fixture in the world of work. This diversity of "Third World" people will bring about a new sense of purpose, mission and behavior for many organizations. As with women, the old stereotypes that equate difference with deficiency need to be reexamined.

As many minorities move into the world of work, organizations will need to be sensitive to unique cultural factors. Much learning will need to occur as new entrants with different values and expectations seek "a piece of the action."

The issue of job assignments is critical to this. If an organization has a client or customer base that is all-white, are minority employees given an equal opportunity to succeed or fail, or, are they relegated to deal with their own people? This has implications for everything from foundation fund-raising to a company's sales territory assignment. For example, a minority worker may not be assigned a certain sales territory because of the discomfort that the employer may feel his clients may be experiencing in dealing with a minority salesman. Such discomfort concerning color or race may exist despite the proven competence of the worker.

All too often a minority employee will comment that he/she is being treated differently because of race. Whether real or perceived, this feeling forms the backdrop for race relations in the world of work. Many minorities still feel that they have to be twice as good as their white counterparts just to get the same job.

Adding the factors of race and sex to the issues facing today's world of work increases the challenges and opportunities for all in the workplace. For traditional workers, it means learning and accommodating to new entrants with different styles, concerns and values. For the new entrants, it means growth, learning and developing the persistence needed to achieve full membership.

It is within the purview of Human Resource Management to take leadership in dealing with these issues. The application of social work skills to this arena enhances the effectiveness of this effort.

SOCIAL WORK'S CONTRIBUTION

The practice of social work is usually looked at in its most narrow sense: a body of knowledge applying to the field of poverty. While this is importantly so, other areas of application should not be ignored. Social work skills can be applied to various settings.

As stated by Pincus and Minahan (1973), social work is concerned with the interactions between people and their social environment. The purpose of social work, therefore, is to:

- enhance the problem-solving and coping capacities of people
- link people with systems that provide them with resources, services and opportunities
- promote the effective and humane operation of these systems, and
- contribute to the development and improvement of social policy.

Given this as a basis of definition, the world of work can be looked at as a rich setting for applying a needed repertoire of skills. The uniqueness of social work is that it combines values, skills and knowledge into practice. The comprehensiveness of social work education prepares a person to be a practitioner, not a philosopher. Philosophy has its place; however, these jobs require a person who is action-oriented and can hit the ground running.

Counseling, group work, research, policy analysis, program development and planning all are social work skills which can contribute to the world of work. The broad field of human resources provides a rich setting to apply these skills. The opportunity for novel ways to practice abounds.

HUMAN RESOURCES CONNECTIONS: THE ARENA

Human Resources has traditionally dealt with the "people" side of the world of work, whether in the public, not-for-profit, or business environment. The terms "personnel" and "human resources" are many times used interchangeably.

"Personnel" typically has to do with the tasks of hiring, firing, payroll and benefits administration. In small organizations, the sole proprietor or chief administrator would perform these basic functions. This was especially true during the turn of the century. As more laws and social legislation were passed, the required knowledge and complexity of the field increased requiring more people to manage these functions. For instance, in 1935 the Congress passed the Wagner Act or National Labor Relations Act which established the principle that employees should be protected in their rights to organize and bargain collectively concerning wages and working conditions. The Taft Hartley Act amended the Wagner Act and forbade a series of unfair labor practices by unions. The Landrun-Griffin Act provided for further amendments governing labor-management relations.

Furthermore, there were other pieces of social legislation bringing about more complexity in the world of work. The Wage/Hour laws governing wage requirements and child labor rights; various Equal Employment Opportunity laws, e.g., Title VII of the Civil

Rights Act, Executive Order 11246, the Age Discrimination Act and the Sexual Harassment Guidelines; the Occupational Safety and Health Act; and various other Federal and State Labor Laws.

The impact of all these laws was to impose requirements on employees to provide for the social protection, health, safety and well-being of the American employee. A residual impact was that the complexity and bureaucracy for administering these laws has increased. This increase also spawned numerous occupational specialties and departmental organizations, such as benefits clerk, compensation specialist, labor relations manager, health and safety coordinator, etc. This resulted in the renaming of the term "personnel" to "human resources," which reflects a greater breath of responsibility and depth of focus.

It is the combination of these forces and factors which provide a target of opportunity for social work skills.

HUMAN RESOURCES AREAS OF PRACTICE

Originally, social workers entered the world of work through Employee Assistance Programs (EAPs). These programs provide an extremely valuable service which enable workers to cope and function more effectively. There are additional areas, however, where social work skills can be instrumental to the success of workers.

One such area is Employee Relations (ER). An ER Manager is concerned with promoting harmonious relations between employees and managers. An ER practitioner counsels, handles employee complaints and resolves conflict. He/she also resolves grievances and administers the disciplinary process. Whether there is a union or union-free environment, the goals of an organization are more effectively accomplished when its members are working cooperatively. The successful working through of conflict, good communications and team/group management skills are essential if this role is to be performed well.

Plans and Benefits Administration is another area where social work skills can be applied. A practitioner here would inform employees of their benefits and resolve various personal issues that arise. For example, an employee may require surgery and needs to understand the level of benefits, deductibles, out-of-pocket costs, etc. A change in a person's family situation such as a divorce or marriage may also require modification of various health coverages.

The area of Equal Employment Opportunity/Affirmative Action (EEO/AA) also can lend itself to a repertoire of social work skills. EEO/AA officers monitor an organization's compliance with the law and develop programs to effectively manage a racially/sexually diverse work environment. Practitioners here also investigate problems of potential discrimination and counsel parties to resolve complaints. Not only is there a need for policy analysis and program development skills, but the ability to counsel and manage conflict as well. The ability to be sensitive to client needs and empower them to more effective levels of functioning is key in this domain.

The Training and Organization Development areas are also receiving increased attention today. Training efforts involve the formal transmittal of skills, information or awareness in a seminar or workshop format. Areas such as communication, time management and supervisory skills are just a few of the topics that can be taught. Courses and programs can be developed to increase the ability of employees to work together.

Additionally, employees need retraining to help them learn new tasks and to increase their ability to perform the job better.

Usually Organization Development (OD) efforts include training, but go beyond it in terms of application. An OD practitioner conducts employee sensing surveys which research how people are feeling and what the morale is in an organization. They will also make recommendations based on their findings. Recommendations may include doing team building; redesigning jobs to provide more variety; developing a career development program; structuring a performance appraisal system; or conducting a goal-setting session.

The functions of Training and Organization Development are key to building an effective workforce and contributing to organizational productivity. Consulting ability and needs assessment skills are of utmost importance in this area. The social work attributes of good communication skills and the ability to separate problems from symptoms are critical assets.

Having a knowledge of research methods, planning techniques

and group facilitation is indispensable to the practitioner who would be successful in Training and Organizational Development.

FACTORS IMPACTING ON SOCIAL WORK CONTRIBUTION TO HUMAN RESOURCES

Given this array of options, how does one consider an area of practice. There are a few factors that guide a person in making a successful contribution to Human Resources. First, the practitioner must decide which job is the best fit for his/her skills, interests and abilities. A person with a clinical bent may find Plan and Benefit Administration boring and unchallenging. On the other hand, if a person enjoys research, EEO/AA may be a good fit for his/her professional inclination. Just as people lean towards one area or another in social work, the same inclination will guide their choice in Human Resources.

Another set of factors has to do with what can be called "industry knowledge." Whether one is working in the union, public, not-for-profit or business sector, knowledge of the playing field is crucial. Preference for working in one industry over another is also a prime determinant of career choice.

One other question that always arises has to do with real or perceived value conflicts in pursuing certain human resource management positions. Do I stop being a "social worker?" Am I coping out of the profession? Is this relevant to the "poor?" Am I becoming anti-labor and pro-capitalist?

There are a myriad number of opinions on these issues. Practitioners should be guided by the code of ethics and principles of the National Association of Social Workers, the National Association of Black Social Workers and the Council on Social Work Education. These principles guide professional conduct and provide values which one can rely on.

The question "When do I stop being a social worker," is the wrong question. Individuals trained in law, engineering and psychology all function in one human resource function or another. The training that these professionals get provides the underpinning of human resource management. The critical thinking, skills and values underlying these professions is what makes the field viable.

A lawyer may not practice as such when he/she is functioning as a labor relations manager, however, there is no doubt that legal skills are being exercised every day.

The same applies to the OD practitioner who is schooled in psychology. Understanding behavior and motivation is critical to success in OD. These same points should go for individuals with professional social work training. Social workers can bring a number of skills and abilities to organizational development. Contracting, process interventions, program planning and needs assessment are just a few of the skills that can spell effectiveness in this area.

CONCLUSION

The application of social work skills to human resources can serve to revitalize the way we are managing our most important asset: people.

The skills and techniques that have been so useful in helping recipients of services can be just as useful in helping service-deliverers. If the world of work is to be a vital and worthwhile arena, then human resource management must play a more important role. Employees can deliver more effective services, programs, and products when they are satisfied at the workplace.

Social work can enhance the ability of human resources to improve the world of work. The shift to this new paradigm will require courage, creativity and flexibility.

REFERENCES

Anderson, Howard, J. (1980). *Primer of Labor Relations*. Washington, DC: Bureau of National Affairs.

America, Richard F. and Anderson, Bernard E. (1978). *Moving Ahead: Black Managers in American Business*. New York: McGraw-Hill.

Dickens, Floyd and Dickens, Jacqueline B. (1982). *The Black Manager, Making it in the Corporate World*. New York: AMACOM.

Ferguson, Marilyn. (1980). *The Aquarian Conspiracy: Personal and Social Transportation in the 1980's*. Los Angeles: Houghton Miffin.

Galenson, Marjorie. (1973). *Women & Work*. Ithaca: Cornell University Press.

Harragan, Betty L. (1977). *Games Mother Never Taught You: Corporate Gamesmanship for Women*. New York: Warner.

Matemeyer, Walter E. (1978). *Classics of Organizational Behavior*. Oak Park, IL: Moore.
Pincus, Allen and Mirahan, Anne (1973). *Social Work Practice: Model & Method*. Madison, WI: Peacock.
Schaef, Anne W. (1981). *Women's Reality*. Minneapolis: Winston.
Toffler, Alvin. (1980). *The Third Wave*. New York: Morrow.

Job Loss and the Occupational Social Worker

Brian Foster
Lee Schore

SUMMARY. Economic and technological changes are creating workplace and labor market upheavals. While new jobs are being rapidly created, many old ones are destroyed. Some new jobs are high-paying, but many are low-paying with little opportunity for advancement. Especially affected are higher-paid blue-collar workers and middle managers, often ill-equipped to cope with job-change. The authors discuss the impact of job-loss and downsizing on individuals and organizations, and describe current dislocated worker and outplacement services. Occupational social work skills are seen as particularly appropriate for lay-off interventions.

In the United States, self-esteem, personal well-being and prosperity are intimately tied to stable employment. Today however, during a period of economic restructuring, massive job upheavals are sorely testing the way that our society provides for its members. Moreover, at a time when approximately one employee in twelve faces involuntary job loss every year, the social "safety net" is in shreds, with less than 30% of unemployed people receiving unemployment benefits. This article looks at trends in layoffs, their impact, existing programs for dealing with employee job loss at all levels, and emerging roles for social workers in the field.

Brian Foster, MS, ACSW, is President, Brian Foster & Associates, New York, NY. Mailing address: Brian Foster & Associates, 401 W. 47th Street, Suite 6, New York, NY 10036. Lee Schore, MSW, LCSW Diplomate, is Executive Director, Center for Working Life, Oakland, CA. Mailing address: Center for Working Life, 600 Grand Avenue, Suite 305, Oakland, CA 94610.

TRENDS IN EMPLOYMENT AND UNEMPLOYMENT

Over twenty million Americans (roughly one sixth of the workforce) change their jobs each year, half of them involuntarily. In the years 1981 to 1985—which included periods of both recession and expansion—over 19 million jobs were lost to the American economy while 22 million new jobs were created, a net gain of nearly 3 million (Birch, 1987). The largest corporations (over 500 employees) actually experienced a net loss of 430,000 jobs while small companies (below 100 employees) created a net *increase* of 3.3 million jobs. It is sobering to see a 1988 study by the Joint Economic Committee of Congress (AFL-CIO News) report that the average new job provides $10,000 per year *less* in compensation (pay + benefits) than jobs that are lost.

Summary statistics on new job creation can thus mask a great deal of underlying upheaval in the job market. While cyclical unemployment (recessions) is always likely, and while many people change jobs for personal reasons, we also see growing job destruction (structural unemployment) due to a combination of factors:

Globalization of the world economy. Prior to World War II imports into the industrialized countries, primarily the United States and Europe, were in the form of raw materials that were then turned into consumer goods available domestically and for export. Now, however, high-quality manufacturing takes place in a large number of less developed countries. Goods, rather than materials, are now imported by the U.S. The effects of this process are to eliminate manufacturing jobs and reverse the balance of trade.

Overvalued U.S. dollar in the 1980s. Exchange rate movements pushed the dollar high in value against other currencies, making imports cheaper and exports more expensive, increasing job loss.

Technological change. Rapid technological change affects blue-collar jobs as automation, robotics and job redesign lower the labor content of the manufacturing process. The widespread use of computers also reduces the need for clerical workers. At the same time, the development of worldwide computer information networks makes it possible to transfer white-collar work out of the country. Because of this more sophisticated technology, many new jobs need a higher level of technological skill, higher literacy levels or better communication skills. At the lower end of the hierarchy, increasingly simplified jobs offer low wages, poor advancement and low social status. Old skills are redundant while new jobs go begging because of the shortage of people with specialized new skills.

Merger-mania. Fierce competition from economic globalization, along with a recently very relaxed anti-trust attitude, have contributed to the frenzy of large-scale corporate takeovers and mergers. They may produce economies of scale, but also may require sale of assets or reductions-in-force simply to pay for the cost of the buy-out.

Middle management "delayering." As a by-product of mergers, business decentralizing and acute cost-consciousness brought on by international competition, there has been a clear effort to reduce the ranks of middle managers in many companies. This particular trend has resulted in still another new population — often middle-aged middle-class males — facing involuntary job change for the first time.

Changing demographics. Currently, 47% of the work-force in the United States is U.S.-born, white and male; however, only 15% of new labor market entrants up to the year 2000 will come from this group (Business Week, 1988). Minorities and immigrants, 17% of the workforce today, represent 43% of its new entrants. Women, currently 47% of the workforce, will comprise 65% of its entrants from 1985 to 2000. As this happens, women, the elderly and minorities will push for greater work and advancement opportunities.

Job instability. As the economy continues to shift from a manufacturing to a service and information base, people are now told to expect to make three, four or five job changes in their lives. Change can provide opportunities, but more likely loss, fear, uncertainty and anxiety. As an employment pattern emerges with frequent job and career changes (and losses of benefits) as well as a more diversified workforce, new services will be needed. Because social work has the potential to integrate the insights of clinical psychology, labor relations, education, organizational development and the sociology of work, occupational social workers are ideally suited to this task.

THE ROLE OF WORK
AND THE IMPACT OF JOB LOSS

Job loss can be readily understood as an economic problem, but the impact of the experience goes much deeper. To work and be productive is a basic psychological need. Work is a central and defining aspect of life and it is through work that identity and self-esteem are often defined. Work is a source of pride, dignity and the independence so prized by Americans. Essential to any successful social work intervention is a solid understanding of the client's work life and work setting (Schore, 1987).

Because of the centrality of work, going through a permanent lay-off, closure or termination may bring on a personal crisis undermining the individual's ability to seek a new job or career. To understand why lay-off can be devastating, it is essential to see it as a profound experience of numerous losses (see Table 1).

Failure of the American Dream. Many workers have structured their lives around the idea summed up in popular culture as the "American Dream." That dream is widely seen as a series of re-

TABLE 1. Losses Suffered by Dislocated Employees

Wages and benefits

Loss of security

The "work family"

Structure for the day

Role as worker and provider

Sense of being productive

Control over life

The ability to trust

The "American Dream"

Pride and dignity

Role in family

Self-esteem

Social status

wards that come from working hard and doing a good job, and includes good pay and benefits, the ability to support a family, a sense of social belonging and economic security. Many American workers have "played by the rules," living up to their part of the bargain in order to receive these rewards. People facing job loss now find that because of new technology and economic restructuring, the rules have changed and they are abandoned instead of rewarded. The perceived failure of the "American Dream" represents a serious psychological loss.

Loss of the "work family." One of the most difficult losses is that of the "work family." In virtually every work setting, informal networks of relationships have been critical social support systems. Often the people at work have been a valuable self-help group, sharing a great deal as they came to know each other in intimate ways. When people are laid off they may be suddenly isolated and must face this most difficult situation without the support of those who have been closest to them over the years. The grief of this loss is another factor that makes it difficult for people to move forward.

Restructuring of daily life. After job loss, people are usually quite unprepared for the disorientation that can accompany the disruption of the daily routine. While employed, the pattern of each day was known but now there is no frame to shape the day. Many people find it very difficult to develop a plan and act on it without some defining routine. Helping a client set up a new daily routine can be an important social work intervention.

Self-esteem. Employees must face fundamental issues of personal identity and self-worth just when many supports are withdrawn. For many people, their identity is strongly tied to their roles as worker, family provider, and as productive citizens. When the objective basis of these roles is stripped away there is a danger of growing depression and anxiety. For men and women alike, job loss undermines their sense of control over their lives.

Impact of job loss on the family. While the employee is the one who gets the termination notice, the lives of family members are dramatically impacted. In effect, the entire family has been "laid off." Roles and expectations that have gone unquestioned during normal times are suddenly challenged. The structure and security of the family may be shattered. Roles shift, life-styles may change dramatically, college opportunities for children fade, homes are lost. Family violence and divorce rates rise in direct relationship to mass layoffs and closures (Brenner, 1973). While services — including counseling and support — are often available for those who have lost their jobs, they are seldom available for family members who may be as vulnerable and fearful as the laid-off worker. Providing services to the whole family should be a major goal of social work interventions.

Self-blame. It is surprisingly common for employees to blame themselves for the difficult situation they now face. Even if their plant or department has been profitable and productive, they may blame themselves for not "working hard enough," or "getting too many benefits." Self-blame may also intensify the feelings of shame and guilt at not fulfilling their expected roles. These feelings may be psychologically paralyzing and make it difficult for people to seek help or use it effectively. For this reason services for dislocated workers should make access as easy and as unstigmatized as possible.

Physical and psychological effects of job loss. As unemployment rates rise so do the statistics reflecting mortality, heart failure, alcohol-related deaths from cirrhosis, divorces, suicides, homicides and admissions to mental hospitals and prisons (Brenner, 1973).

Unemployment exposes people at all levels to a wide range of stress-related symptoms. The physical symptoms can include susceptibility to colds and flu, fatigue, headaches, stomach problems, smoking, weight changes, sleeping too much or too little, and high blood pressure. Psychological symptoms may include: an inability to relax, increased use of alcohol and drugs, irritability, apathy, depression, inappropriate anger, increased domestic problems and domestic violence. These symptoms may become serious obstacles to people's effectiveness in coping with job loss, finding new work or using training opportunities.

Groups facing special barriers to employment. As difficult as job loss can be for the individual, there are whole groups that face additional difficulties. Older workers will find themselves faced with illegal, but real, discrimination in seeking employment which may intensify questions of self-esteem and self-worth. Minorities, disabled workers, and increasingly those without high school diplomas and the illiterate face parallel problems. Single parents face childcare problems along with the reality of no second income to fall back on and no one else at home for psychological support.

THE ORGANIZATIONAL DIMENSION OF JOB LOSS

When a mass lay-off is likely, social workers should consider two important factors beyond offering services to individuals; (1) viewing the downsizing organization itself as a client; (2) getting involved in helping the organization make long-term plans. Social workers can seek to have their voice heard at the earliest possible moment—perhaps as advisers to downsizing committees—and be available right through from pre-lay-off programs to the post-lay-off follow-up process.

A well-planned downsizing contains the following elements (Combre and Foster, 1989):

— Ample advance notice to allow people time to adjust
— Perceived fairness
— Clear, honest, timely, full and frequent briefings by management to all staff
— Full involvement of all employees in the lay-off process
— Preparation of managers and personnel officers on appropriate behavior and strategies
— Flexibility of approach in cutting costs, eliminating positions and providing services
— Transition services for laid off *and* surviving employees.

Unfortunately, managers commonly delay action until the last minute and then handle lay-off interviews poorly because of their own discomfort. Managers may also resist advance notice for fear of sabotage or other disruption. Experience shows however that if those directly affected are *not* involved in the lay-off process until the last minute, effects can be much worse than giving early notice.

A sudden and brutal lay-off will also create hostility, fear, cynicism, absenteeism, sickness and low productivity among remaining employees. Skilled people whose talents are sorely needed may "jump ship" and resign. Angry former employees or their unions are more likely to seek redress through the courts. Growing attention is being paid to the shape of companies after they have laid off people since organizations and "work families" go through their own change and loss experiences (Brockner et al., 1987). An organization that pays attention to the proper process of restructuring and the reasonable feelings of its employees while it downsizes can far better rebuild a sense of community and work family. Occupational social workers have roles to play in all stages of this change process (see Table 2).

THE CURRENT STATE OF DISLOCATED WORKER SERVICES

Transition services currently available to laid-off workers may be provided by internal staff, but are usually delivered by private consultants, labor unions or voluntary agencies operating with public funds. As job loss accelerates in the economy, the demand for such services is likely to increase. EAPs traditionally have not staked out a role for themselves in this area although there is potential for them to do so (Combre and Foster, 1989). Occupational social workers need to know what benefits are available and how they can be used to help workers examine their full range of options. The psychosocial work-assessment forms offered in Figures 1, 2 and 3 may be useful in this connection.

Services for Dislocated Blue-Collar Workers

The greatest impact of mass layoffs and closures during the 1980s has been in the blue-collar world of heavy industry. Former Secretary of Labor Raymond Donovan characterized the typical dislocated worker as, "A male, 40 years of age or older, married with teen-aged children, with 20 years of seniority in a job in heavy industry, a union member with good wages and benefits."

Some of these workers have benefits available to them for re-

TABLE 2. Roles for Social Workers in Mass Lay-offs

Consulting and Advocacy
- Representation on change and downsizing committees to provide consultation and advice
- Ensuring that ample advance notice is given and that frequent, honest, and sensitive communication between management and employees takes place
- Preparation of managers, personnel officers and union representatives for the change and lay-off processes
- Advocacy for reasonable termination services for those dismissed including retraining, "inplacement" (internal job-finding), severance, continued benefits, retirement planning, outplacement/job search services
- Advocacy with community agencies and unions for the needs of dislocated workers
- Paying attention to survivors; preparation of managers for group discussions and meetings with staff.
- Educating employers, communities, worker groups and union officials on legal rights, such as advance warning.

Program Planning
- Fundraising ; JTPA proposal writing
- Establishing procedures and links between the EAP, community resources, internal job search procedures and other services to insure effective and accessible case management services.

Training and Workshop delivery
- Developing and delivering workshop materials on outplacement, career planning, life planning, stress management, retirement, relocation and financial planning to complement workshops offered by other specialists.

Individual and Family Counseling
- Supplementing and following up on other services already provided during the downsizing or closure
- Providing family counseling, usually overlooked for mid-level and hourly employees
- Linkingthe EAP and other service providers for comprehensive case-management and targeting at-risk individuals.

Organizing and Facilitating Support Groups
- Self-help groups and Job Clubs

Community Relations
- Helping bring employer, community agencies, union and other groups together to maintain employment or buffer the effects of lay-off for the community

Legislative and Social Action
- Encouraging the community and governmental agencies to open up employment opportunities for the laid-off group, to buffer the effects of future layoffs and to provide ongoing services.

A: EMPLOYEE SKILLS AND SUPPORTS

Who can you count on for support while you are unemployed?
        name   kind of support
_____   _____
_____   _____
_____   _____
_____   _____
_____   _____

What stressful relationships are you facing?
_____
_____
_____

What changes have you noticed in your family since the lay-off?
_____
_____
_____

Have you ever had job or vocational counseling before?
_____

When you were in high school/college,
    What did you want to be? _____
    What was your favorite subject? _____

What are you most proud of in your life?
_____
_____

What kind of job/career do you want next? What will be the most
important thing to you in your next job?
_____
_____

What training have you had:
        _____OJT (On the job training)
        _____Apprenticeship
        _____Proprietary/Business School
        _____Community College
        _____College   _____# Credits? _____2 Year? _____4 Year?
        _____Continuing education
        _____Graduate
comments: _____
_____
_____

What other off-the-job training, skills, or hobbies do you have and
enjoy? _____
_____

FIGURE 1. Psychosocial Assessment

B1: WORK HISTORY FOR HOURLY WORKERS
Use one copy of this sheet for each <u>employer</u> that the client has
worked for, identifying different jobs and promotions <u>within</u> the
same company on the same form. Start with the latest employer and
position, and work backwards.

WORK EXPERIENCE:
Name of Company: _____
Address: _____
Employment dates: started_____ final day of work _____
Final wage_____per hour
Reason for leaving: _____
Describe major duties, and skills on the job: last job and
department, and date started there: _____
_____
_____
previous job and department, and date started there:
_____
_____
previous job and department, and date started there:
_____
_____
previous job and department, and date started there:
_____
_____
Union and address:_____
Did you have any grievances? What happened to the
grievance(s)? _____
_____
How often were you laid off with this company?
_____
What Benefits do/did you have from the job?   expiration dates
_____Health Insurance:self   _____
_____Health Insurance:family   _____
_____Dental/Eyeglass   _____
_____Prescription Drugs   _____
_____Pension   _____
_____Childcare/Eldercare   _____
_____Severance Pay   _____
_____ESOP*   _____
_____College/Training Tuition   _____
_____S.U.B.+   _____
_____Trade Adjustment Assistance _____
_____Disability Insurance   _____
_____Workers Compensation   _____
_____Recall Rights   _____
_____Relocation Help   _____
_____Credit Union   _____
_____Profit-sharing plan   _____
_____Other: _____
  * Employee Stock Option Plan   + Supplementary Unemployment
                                   Benefits

FIGURE 2. Psychosocial Assessment

B2: WORK HISTORY FOR SALARIED WORKERS
Use one sheet for each employer that the client has worked for,
entering different jobs and promotions within the company on the
same form. Start with the latest employer and work backwards.

WORK EXPERIENCE: Start with the last position :
Name of Company: _____
Address: _____
Employment dates: started_____ final day of work_____
Final salary $_____ per week? fortnight? month? Bonuses?_____
Reason for leaving: _____
Describe major duties, and skills on the job: last job and
department, and date started there: _____
_____
_____
_____

previous job and department, and date started there:
_____
_____

previous job and department, and date started there:
_____
_____

previous job and department, and date started there:
_____
_____

Have you been through a lay-off, major restructuring or downsizing
before ?

What Benefits do/did you have from the job?   expiration dates
_____Health Insurance:self   _____
_____Health Insurance:family   _____
_____Dental/Eyeglass   _____
_____Prescription Drugs   _____
_____Health/Fitness program   _____
_____Childcare/Eldercare   _____
_____Pension   _____
_____Severance Pay   _____
_____ESOP* Stock Options   _____
_____401(k) plan   _____
_____Credit Union   _____
_____Profit-sharing plan   _____
_____College Tuition   _____
_____Disability Insurance   _____
_____Outplacement   _____
_____Inplacement(Competitive Rehire)_____
_____Relocation Help   _____
_____Career Center/Office use   _____
_____Other: _____
   * Employee Stock Option Plan

FIGURE 3. Psychosocial Assessment

training and outplacement to buffer the effect of the closing; many do not. Most workers still have little or no advance notice of closures and receive only six months unemployment insurance by way of extended benefits. In some layoffs, medical benefits are extended for a few months. The new federal Worker Adjustment and Retraining Notification Act (WARN: effective February 4, 1989) mandates advance notice of closings for some employee groups, although many workers may be outside its scope.

The vast majority of blue-collar workers, and many white-collar workers, receive little direct assistance for the life transition that occurs when they are laid off. In the highly competitive and volatile job market that exists today, these workers—many of whom have not had to look for work for years—are at a great disadvantage. The skills required for competing for jobs are entirely different from those of 20 or even 10 years ago.

To fill gaps in services for blue-collar workers, the federal Job Training Partnership Act (JTPA) has been providing services to dislocated workers through its Title III (amended from July 1, 1989 by the Economic Dislocation and Worker Adjustment Assistance Act). The JTPA has been a reworked and poorly funded version of the CETA programs of the 60s and 70s, channeling money through local Private Industry Councils (PICs) to agencies. Each state establishes its own system for administering JTPA programs; some operate them through their community college systems, but most states operate through the PICs in independent Service Delivery Areas (SDAs) which are convenient regional units. Some projects are plant-specific, while others may be open to broader groups. In addition to state-based JTPA programs, corporations and unions very occasionally fund and operate programs.

In PIC/SDA projects, plant-specific projects and community colleges, the following services are usually offered:

—Job search skill development workshops
—Interviewing skill training
—Resume preparation assistance
—Help in filling out job applications
—Job referral
—Job clubs

— Classroom training or referral

— On-the-job-training placement

In some programs, social services such as support and discussion groups, transportation, child-care and referral to specialized social services are also available to workers. It is through the provision of such services that occupational social workers are highly valued.

An example of innovative social support services can be found in northern California where the staff of the Center for Working Life currently provides on-site counseling in two JTPA programs and facilitates worker support groups. In addition to individual and family counseling, the staff also provide support services, advocacy, help in filling out application forms, resumes and financial planning. These services are integrated into the existing JTPA programs so that they are accessible to all the enrolled workers. Social services are thus destigmatized by their incorporation into programs dealing with the "presenting issue" — help with finding a new job. One method of achieving this is through the participation of counseling staff in all JTPA services such as orientation sessions and job-search workshops. A team approach is reinforced by daily consultations with other JTPA service deliverers.

Services for Terminated
Senior Executives

Such services are of course much more extensive than those for blue-collar workers. Professional "outplacement" services, offered by private consultants, grew and prospered in the late 1960s on the first wave of post-war corporate downsizing. In an effort to ease the pain and embarrassment of dismissal, as well as to inhibit lawsuits, companies arranged for executives to be counseled in addition to the usual "golden parachute." Paid by companies at a rate of about 15% of the employee's annual salary, this service — delivered by psychologists as well as occupational social workers and other professionals today — endures as the core of outplacement. Counselors provide career, life and job search counseling in the form of:

— Vocational assessment and testing using standard psychological instruments
— Open-ended personal counseling for the individual and his or her family
— Coaching on self-assessment, networking, interviewing and salary negotiation skills, including videotaping
— Resume preparation
— Use of office facilities on the site of the outplacement firm at high-prestige addresses; telephones, answering services, "bull-pen" cubicles or offices and reference books.

Services for Terminated Middle-Management, Professional and Administrative Staff

As the popularity of outplacement services has spread, companies are paying outplacement firms to provide time-limited, simpler and cheaper group services for lower-level staff. Typically, a peer group of 6 to 12 individuals will attend a one- to three-day workshop after lay-off for intensive training in self-assessment and job planning, resume preparation, networking, interviewing and salary negotiation skills. A group session may be followed by limited individual follow-up counseling and the preparation of a camera-ready resume.

Some employers may offer "career continuation" access to job centers, EAPs or office space for a limited period after lay-off, and may also want to offer further training such as career planning, stress management, relocation, financial planning or retirement planning. While outplacement/job-search training is usually valuable, occupational social workers can also suggest and plan these other kinds of training programs and sorely-needed ongoing counseling services. Delivering such services requires "platform" (adult training) skills and sensitivity to individual feelings of loss. Should the employer open an early retirement "window" as a way to avoid layoffs, social workers can be of great help to employees in making decisions about whether to retire or continue working.

Middle-aged middle managers especially face an uncertain future at a time when companies are busy "delayering." Some may face long-term unemployment and an extended job search. Occupational social workers need to be sensitive to these dynamics and offer ongoing support and practical help. Associated problems (e.g., depression, family violence or substance abuse) may be avoided with sensitive interventions.

SPECIAL ISSUES
FOR SOCIAL WORK INTERVENTION

Whichever population is being served, certain common issues must be addressed to enable people to move forward. First, the practitioner must treat the lay-off as a major loss, sensitively helping people and groups through the stages and feelings of their grief at the same time as concrete services are offered. Regardless of whether the intervention is with an individual, a group or an organization, the practitioner is dealing with crisis, shock and frequently massive denial.

The social worker can help people recognize what they are going through, partialize the problems, and allow for systematic decision-making. At the time of this crisis both individuals and organizations may find themselves dealing with a world for which they are totally unprepared.

Second, the crisis is not only the immediate concern of the individual involved but can have a wide and long-term impact on the family, the work organization and the community.

Third, we believe strongly that social workers must be sensitive to the special culture of workplaces, and the problems that their own values may pose in being of service, especially in the areas of race, gender, age and class.

Feelings Over Job Loss

The most critical of these issues will be dealing with feelings that people experience as they face job loss.

Anger

Conventional wisdom suggests that anger is not normally "useful" and should be controlled. During the crisis, managers, personnel officers, union officials (and even social workers) may fear and avoid employees' anger, even though it may well be appropriate. If not properly expressed it can lead to serious problems and be an obstacle to effective action. Validating appropriate anger has a calming effect that allows people to move on.

Fear and Anxiety

Job loss represents a major disruption in people's lives that produces a loss of psychological security and requires a major life readjustment. People may eventually move on to a new job that is better and more satisfying, but that cannot be known in advance. Typically, people experience fear and anxiety because the future is unknown.

There is, however, another reality for many people: many of the new jobs that are being created in the economy are lower-paying and have poorer benefits. Their fears that change is not necessarily linked to improvement may indeed be realistic. As with anger, validating these fears objectifies them and allows them to be addressed directly. The conventional wisdom today is that unemployment is no longer a problem and that there is general prosperity. However this is not true for many people. In frustration at not being able to help find a decent job for a client, the social worker needs to avoid the temptation of falling back on the common middle-class bromide that "there is a job for everyone who wants one," and then proceed to blame the victim.

Denial

Denial is a very powerful issue that must be addressed head-on. Prior to the closure people will believe that "something" will happen to keep the plant or business open. All sorts of rumors proliferate and are accepted uncritically. People will not use available services and benefits because to do so would be admitting that there was a reason to do so. However since denial carries with it a hidden burden of stress, it is critical to identify this pattern and to help people overcome it.

Understanding the Culture of Work

The social worker needs to assess thoroughly the role of work in clients' lives — an area often neglected in their professional training — and what it means when that work is lost. A good assessment will look at the employer, the benefits it provides, its "culture," its "language," its history and the state of employee morale. Where there is a union it is important to explore what its role and history have been, what support and services it provides and what it has meant in employees' lives.

Self-Help

The workplace provides many natural structures on which to build a strategy of choice; the self-help group. Working people are used to coping and have many strengths and successes in their lives but face a short-term crisis of confidence. Rapidly established self-help strategies such as job-clubs, group training or ongoing support networks are an effective and forceful way of reaffirming people's strengths and reconnecting them to their peers after lay-off. An intervention strategy for mass lay-off may include keeping the softball team or the annual dance alive.

Recognizing Differences

To work effectively it is essential to be alert to cultural, ethnic, gender, class and age issues. Exploring an individual's attitudes toward work and its loss will steer social workers away from unconsciously imposing their own values and making poor decisions about what is desirable for the client.

As examples, gender and age may affect attitudes significantly. Women who have entered the workforce later in their lives may cherish the independence that work brings while younger women may view work simply as an unavoidable fact of economic life. Older men may be uncomfortable relying on a wife's income, feeling intensely that it is their responsibility to provide for their families; younger men may welcome their spouse's career and earnings as a way of maintaining their life-style.

Men may well have a habit of "going it alone" rather than seeking help. There are stories of men afraid to tell their families about losing their job, leaving home every morning and returning at a regular time each evening to hide the fact. Such intense and unshared pressure may make it harder for them to secure new work, and worsen the eventual crisis when the job loss is revealed.

ROLES FOR SOCIAL WORKERS

Social workers are trained to intervene at the point where the individual and the environment interact. This systems approach is very appropriate for the world of work, particularly when people experience job loss as a major crisis. Using the unique perspective offered by the discipline, occupational social workers can be instrumental in helping employers, unions and service-delivery agencies design and implement a variety of programs (see Table 2). Programs can draw upon the entire range of an occupational social worker's skills, from individual and family counseling, through group work, training, program planning, organizational consulting, community organizing and even legislative action.

Social workers need to take the long view of the organizational upheaval involved in job loss, especially if massive or sudden. Early intervention pre-lay-off programs should include information about outplacement and retraining options, small group discussion and individual planning sessions. Group discussions are a vehicle for familiarizing people with their benefits and the various career options they face, while at the same time creating a social support environment to help them face issues of denial, anger, fear and anxiety. Individual sessions are used to develop a plan for each worker, whether they are seeking employment, training or education. This is a chance to assess obstacles to employment that will need to be removed for successful reentry into the labor force. Pre-lay-off services are a preparation for readiness to use post-lay-off services which include job-search workshops, resume development, career planning, job placement and retraining, retirement planning, ongoing support groups and individual and family counseling.

Where possible, social workers should use their position to advocate for a broad interpretation of services and for extending to all employees some of the lay-off benefits routinely afforded managers.

Since much of the population that is now in need of occupational services is quite different from traditional social work clients, new approaches—such as those outlined above—need to be implemented, integrating clinical insights with the very practical tasks facing the unemployed worker (Briar, 1988). Such programs should be seen especially as having an important preventative functions. Unemployment rates—particularly long-term—are linked to increased alcohol and drug use, and higher rates of crime, domestic violence, divorce and homelessness. If people start to receive the comprehensive services they need at an early stage of this transition, the burden on family and welfare agencies, shelters and probation officers is reduced.

CONCLUSION

The world of work, once a haven of stability for the majority, is now churning. This challenge extends to the field of social work which must provide services to a new population. Occupational social workers have a responsibility to raise the consciousness of organizations and public alike about the critical role of work in people's lives and the need to intervene when work is lost.

These upheavals also raise broad policy issues. How work is designed, what protections are provided for workers during their employment and after it, and the extent to which social insurance is bound up with employment, are key questions for the social agenda. Interventions by social workers in the workplace, especially during the crisis of job loss, draw upon a wide variety of skills. From legislation through community action, organizational change, training, group work, and interventions with hurting individuals, the world of lost work offers a great professional challenge.

REFERENCES

AFL-CIO News, September 10, 1988.

Birch, D. (1987). *Job Creation in America*. New York, NY: The Free Press.

Brenner, H. (1973). *Mental Illness and the Economy*. Cambridge, MA: Harvard University Press.

Briar, K. (1988). *Social Work and the Unemployed*. Silver Spring, MD: National Association of Social Workers.

Bridges, W. (1986). "Managing Organizational Transitions" in *Organizational Dynamics*. Summer, pp. 34-45.

Brockner, J., Grover, S., Reed, T., DeWitt, R., and O'Malley, M. (1987). "Survivors, Reactions to Layoffs: We Get By with a Little Help from Our Friends." *Administrative Science Quarterly, 32*, pp. 526-541.

Business Week (September 19, 1988). "Human Capital." p. 100.

Combre, J. and Foster, B. (1989). "Downsizing and the EAP" in *Employee Assistance: Programs for the Future*, eds. Danto E. and McConaghy R. Paramus, NJ: Prentice-Hall — forthcoming.

Schore, L. (1987). "The Mental Health Effects of Work: An Issue for Social Work Education," *Catalyst, 21,* pp. 43-50.

Social Workers' Role in Promoting Occupational Health and Safety

Beth M. Lewis

SUMMARY. Workplace safety and prevention of on-the-job illness and injury is an area of concern to all workers and their families. Effective practice with individuals, families, groups and community organizations must integrate an awareness of the historical, social and political dimensions of the field of occupational health and safety with assessment and treatment of psychosocial problems emanating from hazardous workplace and environmental conditions.

INTRODUCTION

The field of occupational health and safety is a broad one, with several academic disciplines, professions and other policy-setting sectors of society all sharing in the activities of research, proposal and implementation of solutions to the problem of workplace and environmental hazards. Throughout the century, the impact of the industrialization process in American society, with its accompanying new forms and methods of production, has necessitated the development of standards of health and safety, involving, as well, the combined perspectives and participation of public health and labor activists.

The social work profession, historically, has played a significant role in highlighting the psychosocial impact of health and safety issues on workers and their families. Beginning in the early 1900s

Beth M. Lewis, MSW, CISW, is a social worker at Yale-New Haven Hospital, and is Assistant Clinical Professor of Social Work in Medicine, Yale University Occupational Medicine Program. Mailing address: Medical/Surgical Social Work—Rm. 5-437, Yale-New Haven Hospital, 20 York Street, New Haven, CT 06504.

with the investigatory work of the social survey movement, pioneers of the profession sought to document the need for social reform measures to compensate victims of workplace injury (Eastman, 1910). Ultimately, by the third decade of the century, members of the profession advocated increased worker involvement in the organization of the workplace (encompassing standards of health and safety) as a means of prevention (Rosner & Markowitz, 1987), alternatively proposing the institution of case management methods in the rehabilitation of injured workers as well as in the system of compensation for family members of workers who suffered disability or death as a result of unchecked industrial hazards (Perkins, 1921).

The health and safety of workers is a pervasive issue in current-day professional practice. Given the magnitude of a problem which potentially affects millions of individuals and families in today's workforce, social workers in a variety of industrial and health-related settings may encounter client situations complicated by occupational health and safety issues. The work of the early reformers continues to serve as a model for practice with an ever-changing workforce; accordingly, a range of direct service modalities—including psychosocial assessment and evaluation at intake, ongoing individual and family casework, and therapeutic and psychoeducational group treatment (both individual and multi-family in membership)—have been developed in the context of the author's work as a member of an interdisciplinary team of health and safety professionals. Community organizational efforts aimed at developing self-help and advocacy groups for the work-injured and disabled have also been utilized, along with outreach and education to the labor and industrial community and its social service network, contributing to the expansion of clinic services to meet identified needs of the industrial community.

This paper will address the role of social work in the field of occupational safety and health, utilizing a model of service delivery developed by the author over a period of eight years in an occupational health care setting. It will combine historical overview of the field—including discussion of current policy as it impacts on practice—with case examples, offering the reader an opportunity to apply knowledge of issues and practice techniques to work with the occupationally ill or disabled population presenting in similar or related settings.

HISTORICAL OVERVIEW

At the turn of the century, when rapid technological changes in work processes together with the absence of legislated protections placed the industrial (largely, immigrant) workforce at risk for death, illness and injury, the United States had the worst industrial health and safety record in the world, with the American worker being two to three times as likely to be killed or injured as their European counterpart (Rosner & Markowitz, 1987). This was the era of the "settlement house,"—a movement of social reformers composed of founders of the social work profession who joined ranks with labor and public health activists, segments of the business and wider communities in an effort to bring about needed change in the deteriorated working and living conditions of industrial areas.

The passage of protective legislation, including the enactment of workmen's compensation, was largely dependent at this time on data compiled through large-scale social investigations, the most notable among which was the six-volume *Pittsburgh Survey* (Kellogg, 1910-1914). The second volume, entitled "Work Accidents and the Law," looked at employer-initiated patterns of compensation for over five hundred workmen injured on-the-job in Pittsburgh in the year 1907, concluding, "that only a small proportion of the workmen injured by accidents of employment and the dependents of those killed get substantial damages" (Eastman, 1910). Parallel development in the field of occupational medicine under the direction of Alice Hamilton, who conducted her initial investigations of industrial workers under the auspice of Jane Addam's Hull House, placed major emphasis on documentation of health risk, disease and the social impact of work-related deaths and disability in selected industrial areas. Hamilton's work furnished the data necessary to pass legislation providing for mandatory medical surveillance of workers in the "poisonous trades" (Hamilton, 1914).

The infamous "Triangle Fire" tragedy of 1911—in which 146 women workers were killed trying to escape the Triangle Shirtwaist

Factory—served as an impetus for the formation of the New York State Industrial Commission. Appointed to the Commission was Frances Perkins, a social worker and witness of the Triangle Fire, who later, as Secretary of Labor under Franklin Roosevelt, led the movement for passage of protective labor laws, ranging in targets of concern from enactment of the minimum wage to standards of workplace safety. Under Perkin's leadership, the New York State Workmen's Compensation Bureau instituted an "aftercare unit," staffed by trained social caseworkers. The function of this unit was to support the capacities of individuals and family members in their efforts to cope with the economic, social and health effects of work-related disability or death. Speaking before the National Conference of Charities in 1921, Perkins cautioned against the tendency to view these services as dispensable during a period of cutbacks in the Bureau:

> The after-care workers have done much to humanize the work of the commission. It is having a setback just now in New York State, and this work will be dropped or curtailed, I hear. It is false economy, and before many months have gone by the insurance companies, the trade unions and the claimants themselves will recognize it as false economy, and the politicians will then realize it is false economy. (Perkins, 1921)

In another chapter in the struggle to promote occupational health and safety, social reformers Grace Burnham and Harriet Silverman were later joined by social worker Charlotte Todes Stern in their efforts to create the Workers' Health Bureau of America, beginning in 1921, and disbanding in 1928—a period generally regarded as the most repressive era in American labor history (Rosner & Markowitz, 1987). The perspective of the Bureau ran counter to the prevailing views of public health professionals at this time who posed safety and health as a technical/engineering problem. Echoing and expanding on Perkins' views on advocacy, Burnham and Silverman saw the Bureau's essential role as strengthening organized labor by providing workers with the data needed to protect themselves from workplace as well as environmental hazards.

In the decades that followed, the social work profession did not remain active within the field of occupational safety and health, as the profession's growing emphasis on individual treatment methods in the agency setting coincided with the development of the industrial health and safety professions — including hygienists and physicians — who gained a firm foothold in the field. The practice of employing company physicians, nurses and engineers, as a means of controlling workplace hazards — as opposed to reorganization of the workplace — became widespread, through the 30s, 40s and 50s. In addition, widescale organization of sectors of the industrial workforce into labor unions brought about the possibility of contractual provisions in the area of safety and health, filling the void in worker protection which had previously been the focus of social reform efforts (Straussner & Phillips, 1988). Organized labor, itself, placed great emphasis on essential ("bread-and-butter") demands, such as wages, working hours, health/welfare and retirement benefits, although organizing campaigns in the more dangerous trades (e.g., construction, mining) continued to have a health and safety focus (Taylor, 1980).

THE FEDERAL OCCUPATIONAL SAFETY AND HEALTH ACT OF 1970 (OSHA)

The passage of the Occupational Safety and Health Act in 1970 (OSHA) represented the culmination of coalitional efforts of organized labor, the fields of occupational medicine and public health, community-based activists and elected officials which had gained momentum through the late 50s and 60s with the passage of legislated protections such as the Federal Coal Mine Health and Safety Act of 1969. The enactment of OSHA provided a mechanism through which the federal government could both formulate health and safety standards as well as enforce these standards in industrial workplaces through the use of on-site inspections and issuance of violation citations.

The OSHAct theoretically combined three essential ingredients of occupational safety and health: (1) A charter of rights and protection for workers; (2) Close monitoring of state participation, and; (3) The framework in which to broaden legislation in order to give appropriate weight to certain health problems arising from the workplace (Taylor, 1980). The Act's federal regulatory function (OSHA) is administered by the Department of Labor, while the scientific/technical research function (National Institute of Occupational Safety and Health, or NIOSH) — theoretically informing the process of standard-setting in the control of hazardous exposures — is administered by the Department of Health and Human Services. The division in the administration of these two distinct but interrelated functions creates problems in implementation of the provisions of the OSHAct — particularly in the area of prevention — and is reflective of the historical separation between the regulatory/preventive and scientific/technical approaches to the problem of occupational safety and health, alluded to in the foregoing overview. Further, experts agree, the realization of OSHA's original mission has been thwarted, during the current decade, due to large-scale cutbacks in the inspection staff, the exemption of certain workplaces (employing a total of over 13 million workers) from OSHA inspections, and the elimination of inspections based on workers' anonymous reports of alleged hazards, in favor of those initiated by reports of imminent danger (Gold, 1984).

CURRENT DIMENSIONS OF THE PROBLEM

Occupational disease and injury continues to afflict a significant portion of the workforce each year. Deaths from occupational injuries currently number about six thousand/year, or about twenty-five deaths each working day (OTA, 1985). In 1982, NIOSH compiled a list of the ten leading work-related diseases and injuries (not listed in order of prevalence): Occupational lung disease; musculoskeletal injuries; occupational cancers (other than lung); cardiovascular diseases; disorders of reproduction; neurotoxic disorders; noise-induced loss of hearing; dermatologic conditions; psychologic disorders; and injuries resulting in amputations, fractures, eye loss, lacerations and traumatic deaths (MMWR, 1984).

Data on work-related disease is available only in fragmentary form, as there exists no accurate and reliable tracking method of occupational disease to date (U.S. Congress, 1984). Three factors which contribute to the incomplete recording of occupational illness are: (1) Many occupational diseases are indistinguishable from nonoccupational illness (e.g., cirrhosis produced by exposure to chlorinated hydrocarbons is indistinguishable from cirrhosis caused by alcoholism); (2) The occupational causes of diseases are often not recognized by employers and employees, as well as by physicians, and; (3) Diseases with long latencies, such as occupational cancers, often occur after employment exposure has ceased.* Recent estimates suggest there are two million workers severely or partially disabled from occupational disease—one-third of whom suffer long-term total disability—390,000 new cases of occupational disease each year, and 100,000 annual deaths (OTA, 1985).

However, these figures may tend to obscure the fact that workers in some industries have borne, and continue to bear, a disproportionate amount of risk for occupational disease. For instance, a total of 100,000 former asbestos workers are expected to die of lung cancer and a total of 70,000 more will die of other asbestos-related diseases. One hundred thousand miners are afflicted with black lung each year and 4,000 will die from the disease each year. Six thousand uranium miners develop cancer as a result of radioactive exposures.

While portions of the workforce may be the beneficiaries of increased access to information about workplace and environmental exposures, workers in the more dangerous jobs may have neither the means to acquire such information nor the ability to take a proactive stance with regard to potential hazards. Low-income workers, who may suffer high rates of injury and occupational disease are, in addition, more likely to experience the effects of decreased access to the health care system at a time when health care needs have been intensified by the reduction in preventive health programs and their often highly toxic environment (Bale, 1984). Further, it has been documented in at least one report that Black and Latino workers are underrepresented in professional jobs in major U.S. cities (Stafford, 1985) and overrepresented in the most dan-

---

*Thus, the Bureau of Labor Statistics' annual survey estimate of 106,000 cases of occupational disease in 1983 consists mainly of diseases, such as acute dermatitis, that are easily diagnosed and readily traced to workplace exposure. Serious diseases—respiratory and neurologic disorders and cancers—are not generally captured in BLS records.

gerous jobs in the hazardous trades (Davis, 1980; Brown & Scheier, 1981; Robinson, 1984). Thirteen to fifteen percent of Black and Latino workers are unable to work any longer due to partial and permanent disabilities caused by their jobs, compared to eight-ten percent of white workers, and face a twenty percent greater chance than whites of dying from job-related injuries and illnesses (Davis, 1980; Coling, 1985). Recently-arrived immigrants, lacking resources with which to choose other alternatives, may face the prospect of working in small, unorganized shops, where information regarding on-the-job hazards and/or protection may not be easily accessible (Friedman-Jimenez, 1988).

SERVICES FOR WORKERS
EXPOSED TO OCCUPATIONAL HAZARDS

In the absence of comprehensive standard-setting and enforcement of existing regulations of workplace and environmental toxins, as well as lack of societal commitment to full employment, portions of the workforce and community residents with such exposures may elect to utilize health services as a means of addressing problematic workplace and environmental conditions. These individuals often seek relief from symptoms as well as opportunities for relocation in employment or residence and financial compensation for losses incurred as a result of changes made necessary by the health problem. Frequently, the social worker practicing in the industrial or health setting may encounter occupational illness without recognizing it as such. Such workers need to be able to recognize the possible occupational etiology of problems and assist with patient and families' efforts to accept and cope with the effects of illness and disability, secure benefits for workers unable to continue at their present job, effect changes in the workplace, where appropriate, and access rehabilitative services and vocational training if disability precludes a return to former employment.

Many factors effect workers' emotional reactions to exposures, including the physical effects of such exposures, personality characteristics, family and social group dynamics, and job satisfaction or dissatisfaction. Factors which have been identified as associated with occupational stress—including the presence of physical hazards—have been associated with psychosomatic symptoms (Report, 1984) as well as with difficulties in workers' adjustment to work-related illness and disability (House, 1980). Other common job conditions which have been identified as "stressors" include: Lack of control over decision-making; lack of opportunity to use skills and intelligence; routine, repetitious work; machine-paced work; shift work; conflicting job demands; excessive or strict supervision; lack of respect on the job; fear of accidents on the job, and; racial or sexual discrimination and harassment (Back, 1981). Stress emanating from workplace conditions has been described as the result of increasing demands coupled with lack of individual control (Karasek, 1979). It has been suggested, therefore, that individual treatment may not be the optimal method of addressing problems created by stressful working conditions (Donovan, 1987), with information and/or consultation to workers, their representatives and employers regarding workplace stressors, their effects on workers, and recommendation of changes, offering workers potentially greater support in the area of coping with occupational stress.

Inadequacies of the present benefit system—notably workers' compensation—designed to subsidize workers and their families who experience loss of income as a result of workplace injury, disability or death, have been documented in the social work literature (Shanker, 1983; Buchan, 1986; Lewis & Mama, 1987). Data gathered by the Department of Labor indicates that Workers' Compensation benefits reach only a small proportion of persons whose deaths and disabilities are attributable to chronic occupational diseases and that a sizeable share of the occupational disease costs are absorbed by the victims themselves and their families (Brown, 1988). An array of disincentives exist to filing for compensation for occupational disease which is not totally disabling, and/or of unclear etiology. While the National Labor Relations Act prohibits employers from firing workers for filing compensation claims, the fear of reprisal from employers has been so widely documented as a disincentive to filing that statutes have recently been instituted in some states which prohibit employers from "harrassing" an employee who has filed for compensation. Such fears of downgrading or job loss, once one has reported an occupational illness to the employer, are unfortunately based on reality, especially in a period of lay-offs. Difficulties involved in maintaining one's level of income while attempting to retrain or transfer job skills to a new, non-exposed setting are also major disincentives for the blue-collar worker. Finally, knowledge that a case will be contested by the employer — as are the vast majority of occupational disease claims (Schorr, 1980) — and the prospect of long months and/or years of waiting for possible benefits, which may end up being denied in the end, also create major disincentives to entering the compensation system (Dunklin & Krieger, 1981). In such cases, social workers often serve as advocates, assisting with access to benefits while also educating patient, family members and collaterals with regard to the strengths and weaknesses of the system, and offering supportive intervention with regard to the impact of unresolved legal issues on social and economic well-being.

Preventive work in this area is limited by the gaps which exist in the knowledge (of both the extent and nature of the problem of occupational illness) and in the failure to implement regulatory policy on the federal, state and local levels. Prevention of occupational disease and injury occurence remains the, as yet, unrealized goal of professionals who, along with labor and community-based activists, some members of the business community, and elected officials, constitute the group of "concerned individuals" (Ashford, 1976) influencing health and safety policy as it impacts on services to workers exposed to hazards in the workplace.

MODELS OF INTERVENTION:
CASE EXAMPLES

Individuals presenting to occupational health clinics for help with medical problems uncomplicated by social issues emanating from the workplace or non-work environment are more the exception than the rule. The assessment phase of intervention with such individuals involves exploration of the work environment, eliciting from the client his/her perception of hazards, relationships in the workplace, attempts to rectify hazardous conditions, and the overall impact of workplace or environmental hazards on physical and emotional health.

It has been suggested that clients' presenting concerns about occupational/environmental health and safety may be divided into the following four broad, often overlapping, categories (Piotrkowski, 1981):

1. Those who are employed in workplaces and/or living in communities where there are suspected hazards and who seek information about the potential health effects of these hazards.
2. Those who have been informed that they have been exposed to health hazards, and are concerned about future effects on health of such exposures.
3. Those with symptoms that may indicate an occupational disease, often seeking further evaluation of work-related etiology.
4. Those with a diagnosed occupational disease, seeking further medical/legal documentation of etiology and/or level of disability, evaluation and treatment.

Workers' and/or Community Residents' Concern About Exposure to Suspected Hazards

Questions about the potential health effects of hazardous exposures comprises a relatively large portion of the concerns presented to occupational health clinics. Such problem presentation may be in the form of individual, family or group expression of need for information and referral to appropriate agencies or professionals, as well as supportive intervention aimed at alleviating anxieties about health effects of exposure, especially where such exposure is ongoing, inescapable, and unaddressed by public agencies. While this presenting concern constitutes probably about one-quarter of the author's clinic caseload, an equally large proportion of the population presenting with these concerns may benefit solely from the information, advice and/or reassurance offered by the occupational health physician and, where appropriate, the industrial hygienist.

Case #1

The leader of a group of community residents contacted the social worker for help with stress related to their concern about the health effects of ongoing exposure to well water possibly contaminated by a nearby toxic waste dump. In this case, residents had already formed a support group and had begun legal proceedings, having retained the services of an environmental lawyer. After first meeting with the lawyer in order to be better informed with regard to the legal and environmental issues posed by the problem, the social worker then met with the group of approximately 12 individuals at the home of one of the members. Prior to the meeting, the social worker had also elicited the group leader's permission to invite a community-based psychiatrist with an interest in environmental and occupational health.

The group members were able to share feelings of frustration about the lengthy legal proceedings, as well as fears associated with physical ailments which they believed may have been caused and/or exacerbated by their exposures, but which physicians had been unable to attribute directly to environmental exposures. The psychiatrist and social worker noted with the group the effect of the lengthy litigation and controversial political context on both the emotional and physical health of members, pointing out how the documentation of etiology can easily become an overriding concern in such a context. Group members felt supported by the intervention, requesting access to the social worker for the future, should similar needs arise.

Workers with Hazardous Exposures

Workers' experience having contact with various known toxins — often, but not always, known carcinogens — may range from daily, ongoing low-level exposure with provision of protective clothing or equipment to unplanned, high-level, unprotected exposure resulting in acute illness.

Case #2

Mr. C. is a 40-year-old truck driver who routinely makes deliveries of toxic chemicals. His visit to the occupational health clinic was prompted by a contact, four weeks earlier, with an "unknown chemical" which he had suspected was hazardous. Since that contact, he had experienced a burning sensation in his mouth which he attributed to having brushed the parcel, containing the chemical, against his face. His attempts to get information about the name of the chemical had yielded resistance from the dispatcher and employer, causing him further concern, as well as anger and frustration.

In the course of the interview, during which he revealed longstanding emotional difficulties related to familial dysfunction and his own past history of alcoholism and psychiatric treatment for anxiety reaction following cessation of drinking, Mr. C. was able to recognize the role that anxiety about the unknown might play in amplifying any symptoms related to the exposure. He also clarified that if he had been given the opportunity to prepare for a potential hazardous exposure, he might have been better equipped to deal with any consequences stemming from the contact.

A referral was made for the patient to follow through with family counseling for acute family problems. Part of the intervention also included having the social worker and physician contact the company and union president to offer guidance in setting up a safety education program for drivers. Reassurance was offered by the physician with regard to Mr. C.'s fears of possible future health effects of the exposure, and he was able to return to his former job, after approximately two weeks. In addition, the union began plans to incorporate a health and safety training program for its regional membership, in an effort to prevent similar occurences in the future.

Workers with Symptoms that May Indicate an Occupational Disease

Emotional strain caused by health problems of unclear etiology may coexist with stress caused by ongoing exposure to a variety of physical and psychological hazards in the workplace. The visit to an occupational health clinic for evaluation of work-relatedness of symptoms may be seen by the worker as an opportunity to share feelings about workplace conditions in the context of professional concern for the possible effects these conditions may have on one's health. Such discussion may, in addition, provide an avenue for discussion of the impact of deteriorating health on work, and family life.

Case #3

Mr. M. is a 38-year-old engine assembler in a large plant where he has worked for the last six years. He is married with two children, ages 13 and 15. Previously in good health, about one year ago he began experiencing numbness, heaviness and weakness in his right hand and recurrent periods of lightheadedness, both at work and at home. Knowing that Mr. M. had ongoing exposure to numerous toxic chemicals at work, his primary physician referred him to the occupational health clinic for an evaluation of possible work-relatedness of symptoms.

In the course of the interview with the social worker, following his physical examination, Mr. M. revealed that over the past few months, the company had required workers to work overtime—sometimes 12 to 16 hours a day—with a note needed from one's physician in order to work the regular 8-hour day. Drug abuse among employees at the plant, Mr. M. said, was rampant. Beyond concern about the effects of toxic chemical exposure, Mr. M. wondered whether these ongoing stresses at work had played a part in the development of his symptoms. He further revealed that his wife, who worked as a personnel secretary in a large firm, was finding it difficult to accept his illness and work disability. Finally, Mr. M. shared with the social worker that he was hoping that the clinic would "provide some answers" with regard to the nature of his problem so that he would be in a better position to plan for the future.

Workers with ongoing or acute exposures to toxic substances may develop sensitivities to exposures at lower levels and to different environmental stimuli from what had previously been tolerated.

Such sensitivities may cause work disability, with accompanying social and economic disruption for workers and their families. Often, laboratory tests may fail to reveal an organic basis for symptoms and, despite documentation of exposures, workers with chemical sensitivities are frequently unable to obtain workers' compensation benefits due to lack of proof of organic dysfunction. Further, the level of exposure causing these symptoms often falls below OSHA limits, resulting in a lack of motivation among employers to correct conditions which do not affect the majority of the workforce.

The psychosocial dysfunction characteristic of chemically sensitive workers may range from relatively mild adjustmental difficulties, to severe disruption in every sphere of interpersonal and social activity. Family members of these workers also require supportive intervention to cope with the consequences of the illness. Individual, family and group counseling modalities may all be required as supportive intervention techniques.

Case #4

Following four successive exposures to high levels of toxic fumes and vapors over a period of three years in his job as a piper in a chemical plant, Mr. L., age 56, experienced loss of smell and severe burning in his chest and throat when exposed to even ordinary environmental stimuli, such as industrial odors from a plant some distance from his home, cigarette smoke, and household cleansers. He was unable to tolerate the workplace environment and work termination was recommended by the plant physician. His family physician also concurred with the recommendation to stop working at the plant. He was finally referred to the Occupational Health Clinic by his union president, for the purpose of receiving further evaluation and documentation of the work-related etiology of his symptoms.

With an eighth-grade education, Mr. L. had little hope of ever achieving the level of economic security he had gained from a lifetime of factory work, and was extremely pessimistic about his ability to retrain in another type of non-industrial job. Initial intervention involved collaborative approaches to treatment, including successive meetings with the L.'s alone and with the physician, union president and vocational rehabilitation counselor, in the clinic, community and union settings. The L.'s also made use of individual and marital counseling, as well as participation in a psychoeducational group for workers with chemical sensitivities, to discuss issues of adjustment to disability, difficulties obtaining workers' compensation and the resultant loss of economic security, vocational alternatives, and the impact of Mr. L.'s work-related illness on the marital relationship. Although initially resistant to psychiatric treatment for diagnosed reactive depression, with supportive intervention, Mr. L. was eventually able to follow through with referral to an outpatient psychiatric clinic in his neighborhood, additionally receiving continued social work intervention during the stressful period pending resolution of his workers' compensation case.

Workers with a Diagnosed Occupational Disease

The cessation of work due to illness, whether temporary or permanent, is a crisis of considerable proportion in the lives of workers, with added significance for those with limited emotional, financial and familial resources. Where there is an established or possible workplace etiology for a presenting medical problem, the relationship of worker to workplace may take on an added dimension of psychosocial stress, as the worker attempts to cope with issues of employer/co-worker responsibility, self-blame and impact on future work opportunity and capability, while, at the same time, dealing with the scope of patient/family adjustmental issues well-known to social work practitioners in health-related settings.

Case #5

Ms. B. is a 30-year-old painter, divorced with one child, age 15. She had developed severe dermatitis as a result of unprotected contact with paint chemicals on-the-job — with OSHA later (after-the-fact) issuing a citation to the company for unsafe work practices. Ms. B. had been able to break into the male-dominated trade two years earlier with the aid of an affirmitive action apprenticeship program targeting women and minorities.

Ms. B. used casework services to discuss difficulties adjusting to illness, involving feelings of anger over the discriminatory treatment of women and minorities which she felt had contributed to her hazardous exposure, as well as feelings of failure for contracting an illness in the course of employment which she had struggled to obtain. In addition to supportive counseling, Ms. L. sought advice and utilized union-sponsored programs offering referral to trade apprenticeship programs, and community resources for women in the trades, eventually locating alternative work in a non-exposed trade.

RECOMMENDATIONS:
THE NEED FOR A MODEL OF COLLABORATIVE
OCCUPATIONAL HEALTH SERVICE

Social work services in occupational health and safety must be carried out collaboratively with the medical and industrial hygiene professions. Environmental modification techniques, beyond accessing resources for individuals and families, involve, as well, the investigation and control of workplace and environmental hazards.

Industry and labor must also be involved at the individual and organizational levels of intervention. Traditional collaborative relationships with physicians in health-related settings must also be strengthened in the field of occupational health care, as the complexity of diagnosis and evaluation of work-relatedness and determination of work disability involves a combination of psychosocial and medical diagnostic and treatment skills.

Diagram 1 is an attempt to illustrate the nature and role of collaborative practice among the professions providing health-related services to occupationally ill/injured workers.

CONCLUSIONS

Occupational health and safety is an area of concern for workers, employers and health-care providers alike. All groups retain a characteristic outlook on the problems associated with maintenance of a healthy work environment, prevention of on-the-job injury and ill-

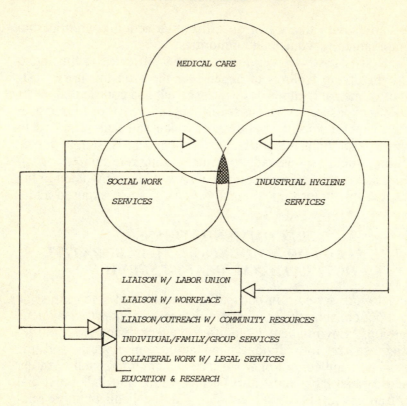

*Middle shaded area of three-dimensional overlap represents collaborative work among the professions in all service activities.

DIAGRAM 1. Model of Collaborative Occupational Health Service

ness, and the aftermath of workplace incidents associated with hazards.

In addition to treating individual workers and their families, the system of occupational health care delivery must, if it is to achieve a stated goal of improving workers' health, incorporate a preventive plan of intervention aimed at changing unsafe working conditions known to have caused or be the potential cause of occupational illness or injury. It must function to effect legislative policy in this area, as well as in the area of benefit systems designed to ameliorate the socioeconomic, medical and vocational rehabilitation needs resulting from workplace illness and injury.

The history of social work practice in the area of occupational health and safety began at the turn of the century, involving early social investigatory work and the introduction of casework methods in work with injured/ill workers, and developing alongside a broadbased movement for improvement of industrial working conditions. Effective social work practice in today's industrial and health-related settings continues to combine an understanding of the social, economic and political factors affecting work organizations and their impact on the health of workers and their families.

Collaborative work with industrial health professionals also involves outreach to industrial personnel and alliance with labor organizations in an effort to promote a healthy work environment. Understanding the role of organized labor in promoting workplace safety is critical to informed practice in clinic and community settings. Such well-informed practice with individuals, families, groups and community organizations is a major component of services provided to meet the fundamental human needs of workers at risk.

REFERENCES

Ashford, N. (1976). *Crisis in the Workplace: Occupational Disease and Injury*. Cambridge, MA: The MIT Press.

Bale, T. (1984). Pain and Plenty: Income Polarization and Health in the 80's. *Health/PAC Bulletin,* 15(4), 5-11.

Beck, A. (1981). *Occupational Stress: The Inside Story*. Oakland, CA: Institute for Labor and Mental Health.

Brown, J., & Scheier, R. (1981). Workplace may be Hazardous to Health of Blue Collar Minorities. *The Chicago Reporter*, 10(3).

Brown, T. (1988). Something Better for Occupational Disease Victims. *American Journal of Industrial Medicine*, 13, 515-518.

Buchan, V. (1986). When the Money Runs Out: Worker's Compensation Woes. *Occupational Health & Safety News Digest*, 2(9), 1-4.

Coling, G. (1985). *Taking Back Our Health: An Institute on Surviving the Toxics Threat to Minority Communities*. Washington, D.C.: United Auto Workers/ Urban Environment Conference, Inc.

Davis, M. (1980). The Impact of Workplace Health and Safety on Black Workers: Assessment and Prognosis. *Labor Law Journal*, 31(12), 723-732.

Donovan, R. (1987). Stress in the Workplace: A Framework for Research and Practice. *Social Casework*, 259-266.

Dunklin, B., & Krieger, B. (1981). *Factors in the Decision to Apply for Workers' Compensation for an Occupational Disease*. Masters Thesis. Univ. of Maryland School of Social Work and Community Planning.

Eastman, C. (1910). Work Accidents and Employers' Liability. *Conference of Charities Proceedings,* 414-424.

Friedman-Jimenez, G. (1988). Occupational Disease Among Minority Workers: A Common and Preventable Public Health Problem. *Occupational Health Nursing*. Publication in progress.

Gold, L. (1984). Worker Safety and Health. In L. Gold, *The Reagan Administration's Record on Labor Law Issues: Report to the AFL-CIO*. 17-22.

Karasek, R. (1979). Job Demands, Job Decisions Latitude and Mental Strain: Implications for Job Redesign. *Administrative Science Quarterly,* 24, 285-307.

Kellogg, P. (Ed.) (1914). *The Pittsburgh Survey: Findings in Six Volumes*. New York: Charities Commission.

Lewis, B., & Mama, R. (1987). The Cost of Filing: Workers' Compensation and Unmet Need in the Work-Injured/Diseased Population. *Social Work Papers,* 20, 30-45.

Morbidity and Mortality Weekly Report (MMWR) (1984) 33/9.

Office of Technology Assessment (OTA) (1985). *Preventing Illness and Injury in the Workplace*. U.S. Congress. 3-26.

Perkins, F. (1921). After-care for Industrial Compensation Cases. *Conference of Charities Proceeding*.

Piotrkowski, C. (1981). Private communication.

Report of the Joint ILO/WHO Committee on Occupational Health (1986). *Psychosocial Factors at Work: Recognition and Control*. Geneva: International Labor Office.

Robinson, J. (1984). Racial Inequality and the Probability of Occupation-Related Injury or Illness. Milbank Memorial Fund Quarterly/*Health and Society*, 62(4), 567-590.

Rosner, D., & Markowitz, G. (Eds.) (1987). *Dying For Work*. Bloomington and Indianapolis: Indiana U. Press.

Shanker, R. (1983). Occupational Disease, Workers' Compensation, and the Social Work Advocate. *Social Work*, 28(1), 24-27.

Stafford, W. (1985). *Closed Labor Markets: Underrepresentation of Blacks, Hispanics and Women in New York City's Core Industries and Jobs*. New York: Community Service Society.

Straussner, S.L.A., & Phillips, N. (1988). The Relationship Between Social Work and Labor Unions: A History of Strife and Cooperation. *Journal of Sociology & Social Welfare*, XV(1), 105-118.

Taylor, G. (1980). The AFL-CIO and Workers' Safety and Health. In Maclaury, J. (Ed.), *Protecting People at Work*. U.S. Dept. of Labor, 209-219.

U.S. Congress (HR98-1144) (1984). *Occupational Illness Data Collection: Fragmented, Unreliable and Seventy Years Behind Communicable Disease Surveillance*.